'The hands that made you, are the hands that heal you'

A Time To Heal

A BIBLICALLY BASED WORKBOOK FOR THE HEALING OF TRAUMA

Dr. Rani Samuel and Dr. Sam Soleyn

First Published 2023 by Dr. Rani Samuel and Dr. Sam Soleyn

ISBN 978-0-7961-4500-0 (Print)

ISBN 978-0-7961-4501-7 (eBook)

TABLE OF CONTENTS

Part One

Part Two

AKNOWLEDGEMENTS

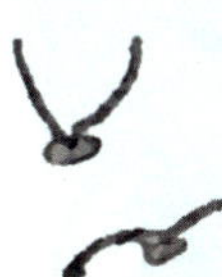
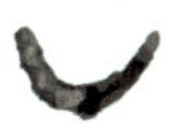

Our sincere thanks to Michael Barrett
for your consistent support and
encouragement with every aspect
of "A Time To Heal", and
your dedicated work in this area of ministry.

Dr. Rani Samuel is a Clinical Psychologist with extensive experience in the area of emotional healing and wholeness. She works in a private practice as a psychotherapist seeing both hospital inpatients and outpatients.

Her work is focused on guiding patients through healing journeys from a place of crisis to one of calm and contentment, in-spite of the storms of life. The processes that her patients embrace deal with both the psychological and biblical aspects of healing.

Dr. Rani is a skilled writer and has written widely on emotional healing. Her books include *Living Stones - Psychological and Spiritual Insights* to inspire, renew and heal your life; *Stepping Stones to Emotional Healing, Pebble Stones, The Healing Emporium* and her debut novel, *In Search of Daniel,* which explores the theme of healing from trauma in the womb. In her books, teachings and conference presentations she shares her professional knowledge

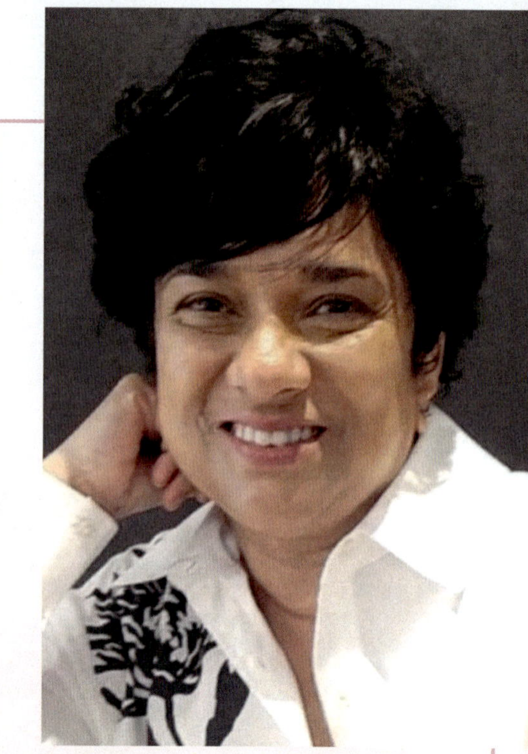

Meet
Dr. Rani

and experience as well as her insights as a committed child of God.

She adeptly blends her psychological competence with pearls of biblical wisdom. Dr. Rani is a spiritual son of Dr. Sam Soleyn. She is passionate about releasing people into the fullness of their divine potential and purpose.

Dr. Sam Soleyn, an apostle whose teachings are recognised internationally, brings understanding and enlightenment to the original intent of God for the creation of mankind. Furthermore, his grasp of the overarching nature of Scripture and of biblical jurisprudence brings clarity to the understanding of the Kingdom of God and its governance. In his book My Father! My Father!, Dr. Sam established the identity of sonship and the principle of 'exact representation'.

Through the restoration of *The Elementary Doctrines* as a foundation for growth and maturity and the re- establishment of the framework of spiritual families led by spiritual fathers, he reveals the order needed to regain the culture of the Kingdom from the mindset of orphans.

Dr. Sam's teachings and the practice of blockage removal provide much needed understanding and relief for many whose souls are trapped in the repeating cycles of depression and despair. Additionally, his messages on the prophetic Scriptures steady believers in the darkness and uncertainty of the present global distresses. The apostolic gifting is most evidently on display in Sam's

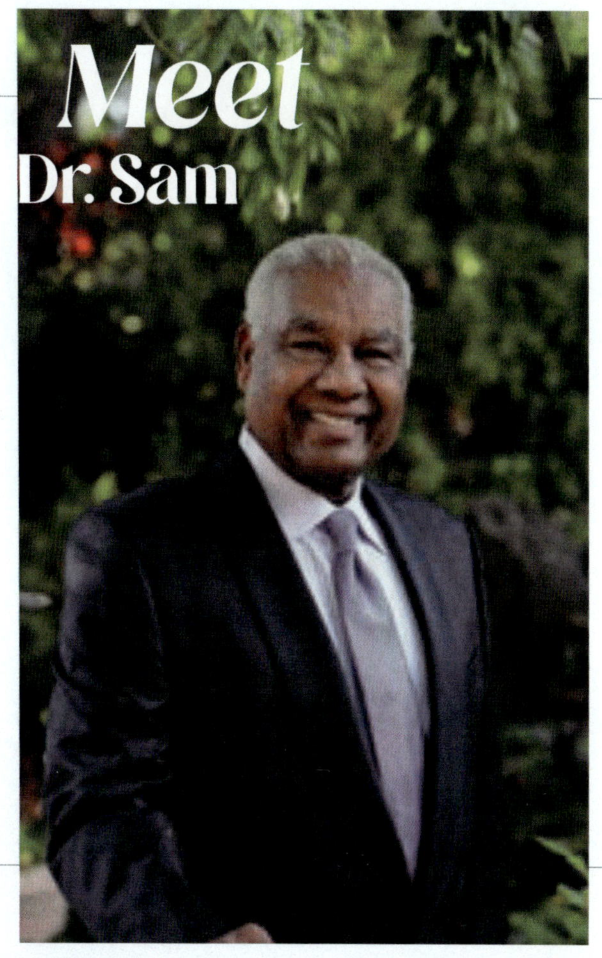

understanding of the unitary whole of the Scriptures and in the revelation of complex mysteries. In his hundreds of messages delivered at conferences and addresses around the world and on television, radio, and the internet, he has brought insights and illumination to audiences for decades.

While relentlessly pursuing the truth, he deconstructs many popular theological positions and challenges many basic religious assumptions. He is known for his boldness, courage, and plainness of speech. His brilliant intellect is as unmistakable as his patience and kindness.

Foreword by Dr. Sam Soleyn

In the creation of mankind, God created a very complex being. He placed this being in the natural world but endowed him with the ability and competence to also live in the spiritual world simultaneously. Accordingly, mankind was given a spirit, a soul and a body. The body houses both the spirit and the soul. The underlying purpose was to produce 'a man in the image and likeness' of God himself.

Such a being would have an eternal purpose that would be developed and matured in the natural realm and within the human body. God gave the human being, a spirit out of His own person to connect the human directly to the mind of God, in the fashion of 'spirit to Spirit'. The human spirit is therefore of the same kind in nature as God Himself.

In this connection, the human would have access to the knowledge, wisdom, and understanding within the person of God.

The human spirit would then inform the soul, which in turn was designed to function in the environment of earth. The vehicle that would facilitate the functioning of the soul is the body. Therefore, the optimally functioning human being would be one whose soul was under the governance of his spirit, and whose actions in the body would put on display the nature of God Himself on the earth.

The order of its operation would be the spirit of man being directly connected to the mind of God; and would transmit to the mind of the soul the intentions of God to be carried out in the human body.

In this fashion, a man 'in the image and likeness of God' would model the character and nature of God within creation. Such a person would be a spiritual person. Although contained within a human form - this spiritual man would display the glory of God's nature in the venue of earth.

Foreword

The first Adam was this prototypical being. However, God always had the final iteration of this man in the image and likeness of God in mind, when he made the first Adam. God had already considered Christ as the final expression of this man. Christ inevitably would be a spiritual man in as much as a man in the image and likeness of God could only be a spiritual man. This was the original intent of God

In the garden of Eden, we are introduced to the enemy of God and man. This enemy with extraordinary skill and cunning, succeeded in separating men from God. In that exchange, the eyes of man's soul were opened and his soul began to act independently of his spirit. Over the many millennia since, man's soul has continued on the trajectory of separating itself from his spirit and acting independently of both the spirit of man and the Spirit of God. Presently, the vast majority of human beings are governed by their souls and are at war within themselves in a conflict between their soul and spirit.

The coming of Christ into the world was God's way of inserting Himself into the lives of human beings. He chose to do so by restoring the communion and fellowship between the Spirit of God and the human spirit. This brought back the soul to its place of submission to the human spirit - thus saving the soul from the control of the Evil One and realigning mankind to God's original purpose.

However, God was not and is not unopposed in this matter. The enemy has grown in both cunning and skill in maintaining the internal conflict between spirit and soul, resulting in man's confusion regarding the central issues of his identity and his purpose.

The major skill of the enemy is his ability to disrupt the human soul, and to cause inestimable distress within the

Foreword

human being by distorting the way that the soul functions.

This creates false identities and profound entrapments, from which it is impossible for the human to escape without the direct intervention of the Spirit of God. When the souls of persons are out of order, people who are highly skilled in their vocations, will often display shockingly erratic behaviours in their domestic relationships - often creating confusion in their spouses, families and intimate relationships. They make it difficult for their close relationships to harmonise these erratic behaviours with the skill and competence those persons otherwise display.

Dr. Rani Samuel has dedicated her life to helping others restore this balance, and to rescue people from the torments of this unreconciled way of living. She has moved well beyond any form of tolerable recovery and

behavior modification into the depths of human brokenness to offer hope and release. I have interacted with her over the course of more than fifteen years and have observed her competence and skill in this healing ministry. She is a trained clinical psychologist whose understanding of the human soul and the attendant brokenness is altogether evident. She is a remarkable resource in the area of understanding the effects of trauma on the soul and the protocols for its healing. This book puts these protocols on full display and is a unique resource for persons seeking wholeness in their souls.

Dr. Samuel is the primary author of this work. It has been my privilege to collaborate with her in producing the final work. Both she and I recognise the invaluable help of our colleague Michael Barrett in developing foundational materials on Blockage Removal from which this book: A TIME TO HEAL draws substantial inspiration.

Dr. Sam Soleyn

Unfolding Healing

Its 4:12am. The sky is a velvety black. A crescent moon levitates alongside two distant stars. It is dawn and in a short while the new day will break. This time between night and day is elusive and it's a wistfully fleeting delight to simply behold the unfolding.

Brushstrokes of silver-grey make an appearance. A hint of amber appears on the skyline and reveals the soft outline of leafy trees and fluttering birds responding to the call of the morning light. There are now golden hues, misty blues and streaks of white light. Slowly, night turns into day and grief written in the sky is covered by a honeyed shawl of hope. Colour has returned to the world.

The unfolding of a morning sunrise is a vivid, kinetic metaphor for the inner healing journey. Watching the cloak of darkness being lifted, and the sun sprinkling diamonds on the horizon, is the picture of hope we carry in our hearts.

Broken Hearts

If your car is broken, you don't spend time repainting the bodywork. If your heart is broken, you don't heal the wounds by concealing them. Many people struggle with emotional pain that is deeply embedded in the past. This unresolved pain manifests in daily challenges such as depression, anxiety, addictions, tempestuous relationships, disease and suicidal thoughts.

We must face the reality of our pain- filled past if we are going to spiritually mature and grow into everything that God intended us to become. In addition, whether you realise it or not, you have a spiritual enemy that seeks to steal, kill and destroy your life. Setting up blockages in the emotions of your soul is the key strategy of the enemy.

"Healing is a journey from darkness to hope"

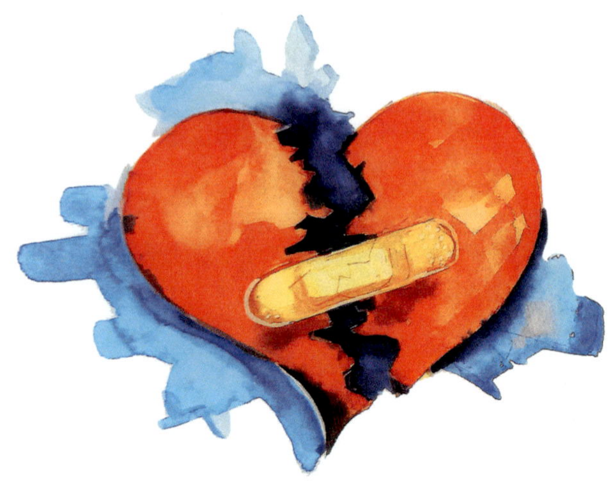

This Healing of Trauma Workbook is the starting-point for dismantling the schemes of your enemy, and accelerating your healing journey. It is designed to help you find your way back to a place of purpose and destiny. This is done by giving you an opportunity to take a deep, candid look at the traumatic experiences of your past, that have left you emotionally scarred in the present. The door to healing and wholeness is opened to you through this process.

How to use this Workbook

Reflective study and writing is a time-honoured practice. This Workbook presents core content and searching questions to guide you on this journey. You are encouraged to pace yourself through each chapter and podcast, in chronological order. Do not rush the process, but be patient, and give yourself ample time to absorb the meaning of the material.

Write out your answers thoughtfully and completely. **You will find that the process of writing them out, will help you gain insights and viewpoints that you may not have known you had.** As you work through the material in this Workbook, you may be surprised at the power of the emotions that come up as you write. This is part of grief processing and recovery, and will move you towards the healing of your soul. Begin and persevere.

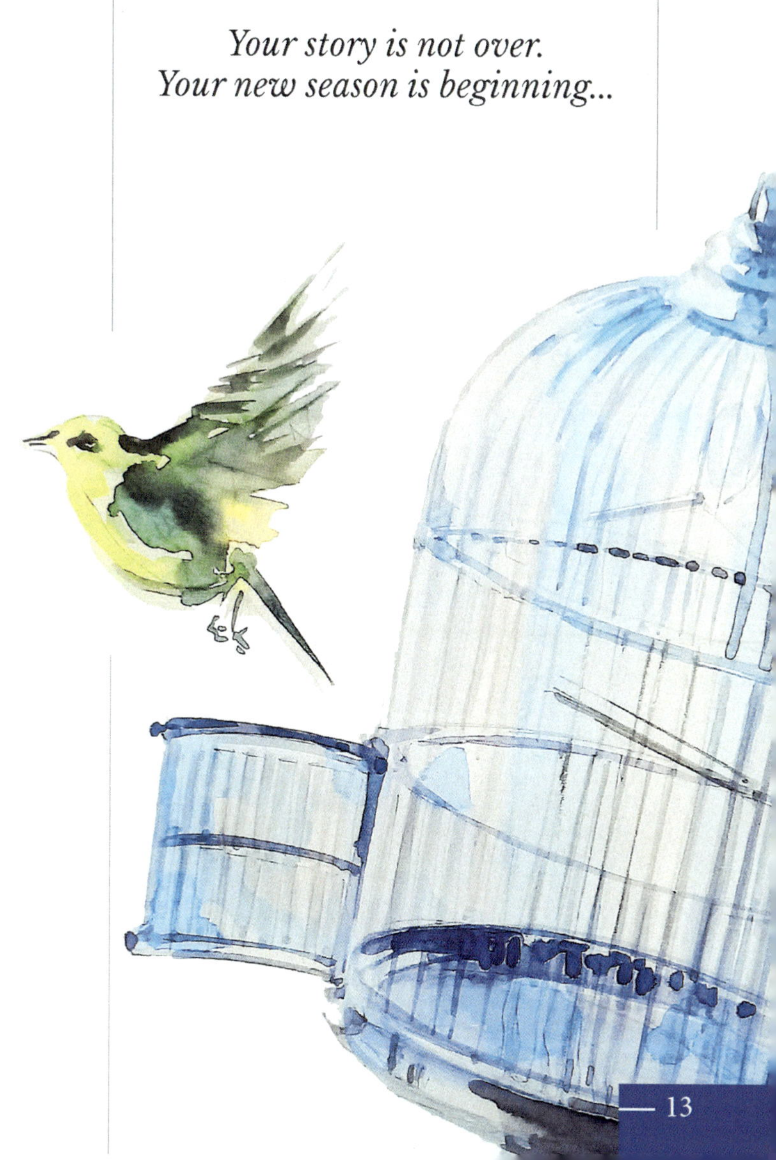

Chapter One

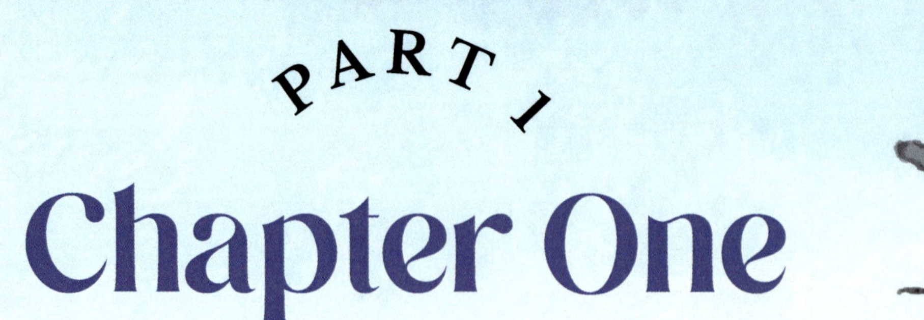

You're Invited

AN INVITATION TO HEALING

*The Hands that Made
You, Are the Hands
that Heal You*

Date: Soonest

Venue: Wherever you are

Time: When you are ready

Dress Code: Come as you are

Healing to Follow

Hideaways for Healing

In early June 2023, I was invited to speak at a church retreat. The campsite was hidden in the sugarcane fields surrounding my home city of Durban, South Africa. I traveled on an open freeway, down a small town roadway and through bumpy sugarcane pathways to arrive at a lush hilltop oasis. Forty people waited in anticipation and apprehension to engage in a weekend of emotional healing. The night before the gathering, I sat quietly and wrestled with how to guide the opening of my teaching session.

The question of how to invite each person into divine surgery challenged me. I knew that no one willingly enters the operating room. The surgeon's scalpel invokes fear - for it will hurt before it heals.

I went before the Lord and asked Him to show me why healing is an invitation from Him. What would He want me to say to every retreat guest and to you also? He led me to thoughts of knitting as artistically expressed in the *Book of Psalms, chapter 139, verses 13-16: 'For You created my inmost being; You knit me together in my mother's womb. I praise You because I am fearfully and wonderfully made; Your works are wonderful - I know that full well. My frame was not hidden from You when I was made in the secret place, when I was knit together in the depths of the earth. Your eyes saw my unformed body; all the days ordained for me were written in Your book before one of them came to be.'*

Hideaways for Healing Continued...

In my clinical practice, patients have spoken of knitting as meditative, imaginative and precise. It's a lost craft to some and a rediscovered art to others. Knitting is also the portrayal of the loving, divine creativity in the womb of our mothers.

As I reflected on this process, my own understanding opened up and I started to imagine two knitting needles, a ball of wool and two hands actively at work. God chose to knit us skilfully in the secret recesses of our mother's womb. It dawned on me that our loving creator and divine surgeon are one and the same.

These supernatural hands heal us when we are broken, bloodied and lying on the floor of life's traumatic experiences. **It's a Holy Surgery.** The invitation to healing involves knowing and trusting that the same hands that made you, now want to heal you - that your Maker is also your Healer.

You do not need to fear God or His methods because He knows your innermost parts and He will restore you to your original sacred blueprint. **God loves you and invites you to let His hands heal you.**

"Healing is Holy Surgery"

Personal Reflection

Healing always begins at the point of acknowledging our traumas and hurts, as well as taking responsibility to enter a healing journey. For many of us, revealing the hidden memories of our past is painful. We go to great lengths to suppress them in order to avoid the emotional pain.

We bury the pain, run from it or even medicate it away. Further, with medical surgery every patient has to sign a consent form to conduct the operation. It's no different with emotional and spiritual surgery. You have to consent to the divine handiwork of God.

> *• What do you most fear about remembering the hurts of your past?*
>
> *• Are you willing to sign the consent form to begin your healing journey?*

Responding to The Invitation

The Invitation to Healing is an invitation to trust God with your wounds. This is the same God who knew you before you were in your mother's womb and engraved a destiny on your spirit.

Write out your response to His invitation to heal you.

What thoughts and feelings (both positive and negative) are brought up as you write out your response?

Thoughts:

Personal Reflection

Personal Reflection

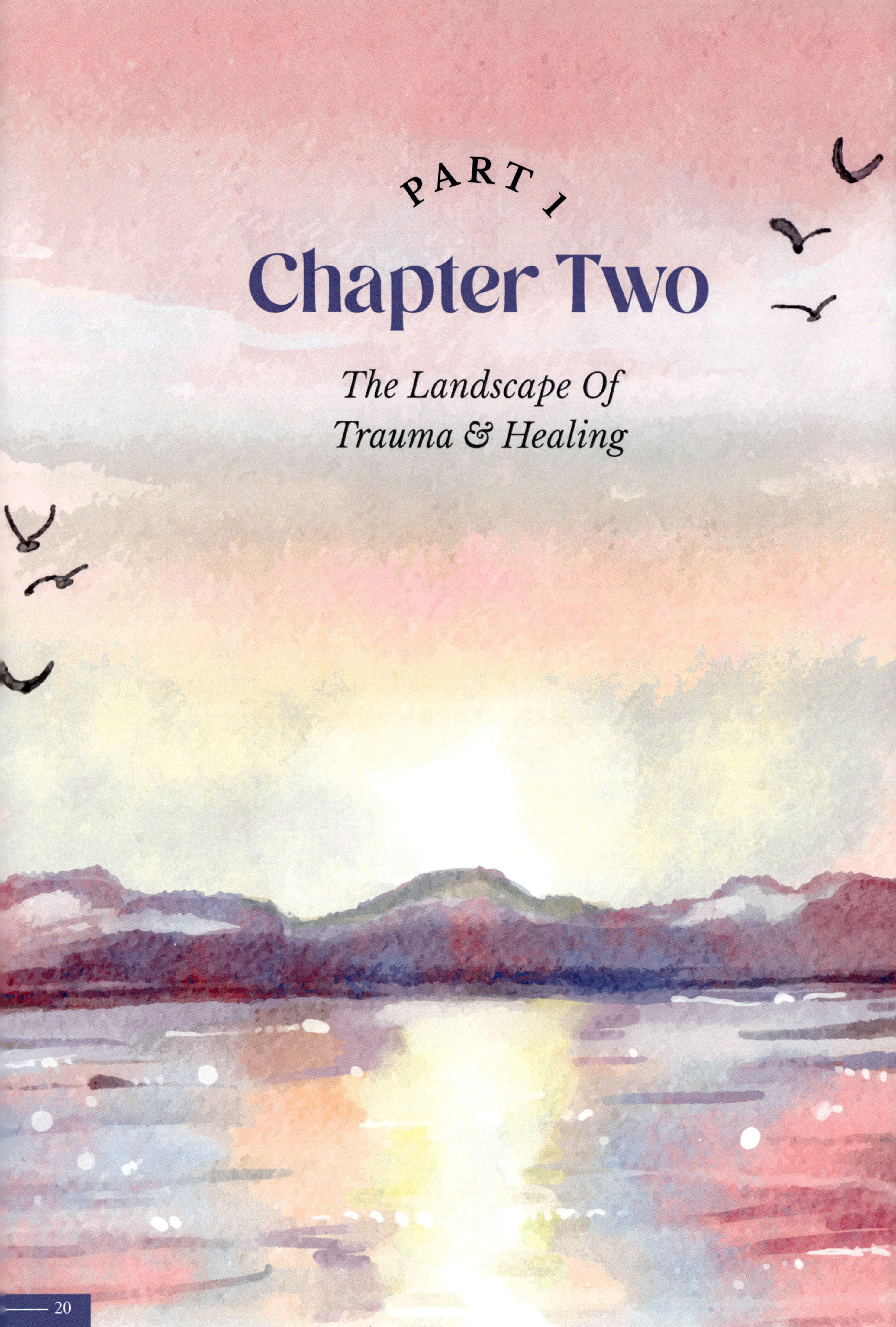

PART I
Chapter Two
The Landscape Of
Trauma & Healing

What is healing?

The word healing has its roots in the Greek word therapia (or therapeuein as a verb) which means 'cure'. It embodies a sense of wholeness and completion. Therapia is the origin of words such as therapist and therapy. An Old English word, haelon, is another word for healing and means to cure and be made whole. The root word of haelon is hal, meaning whole, sound or healthy. Interestingly, hal is also the root of 'holy' and 'hallowed'. **To heal is a holy undertaking.**

What is trauma?

Trauma comes from the Greek word for wound, which can be physical or emotional. This wound usually leaves a scar or imprint on one or more of your emotional life, your biochemistry, your psyche and your body.

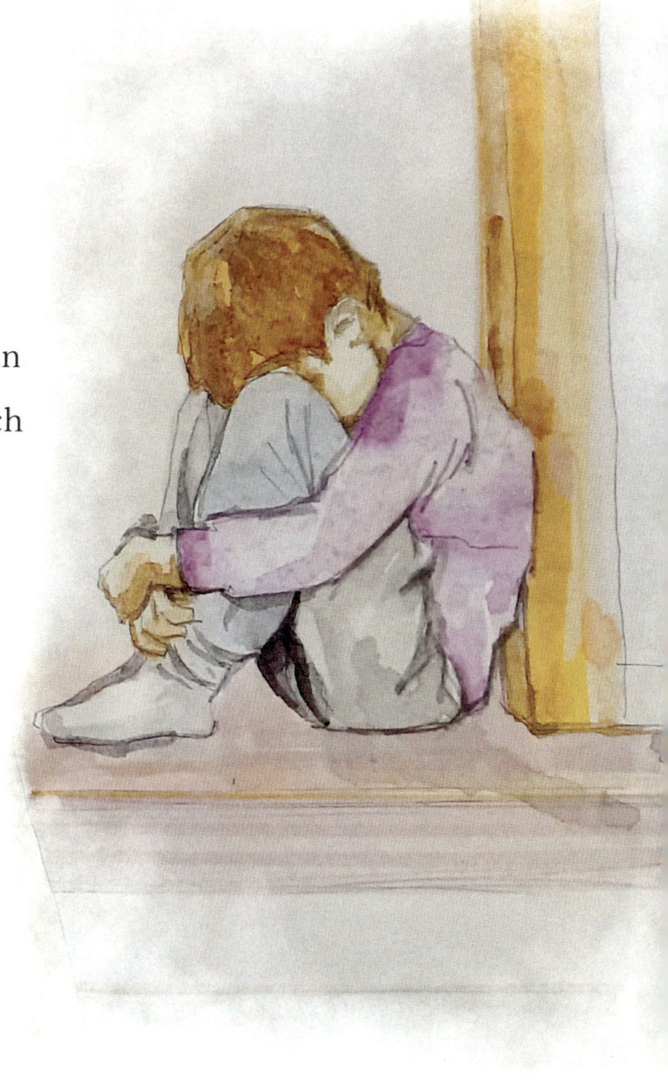

Trauma is caused by external violence which can be physical or emotional. An act of violence such as robbery, rape or physical assault will result in physical wounds as well as emotional.Harsh words, neglect, rejection and abandonment are examples of emotional acts of violence. Our first response to trauma is to attempt to erase it from our minds. There is often a deliberate attempt to eradicate and drive out the traumatic experience from our thoughts. However, trauma refuses to be buried or dismissed.

Understanding Trauma

Healing the Broken-hearted

Every single patient sitting across me suffers from heartbreak. No one can get away from it, even if they try. A broken heart is a wound that needs healing. Heartbreak comes from loss due to death, separation, divorce, a child leaving home or the suffering from wars in our minds and in our world.

My patient Paula is a poet and she was telling me about her grief after the sudden death of her brother in a car accident. 'I am a cocoon of sadness… this small leak of loss in the corner of my heart has turned into a flood in my chest,' she said. 'This heartbreak is silent yet screaming at the same time… it feels heavy, as if my ribcage is tightly packed with small stones that leave no place for breathing. I am simply letting the minutes of aching turn into moments of longing,' she whispered. Paula was at the start of her healing journey.

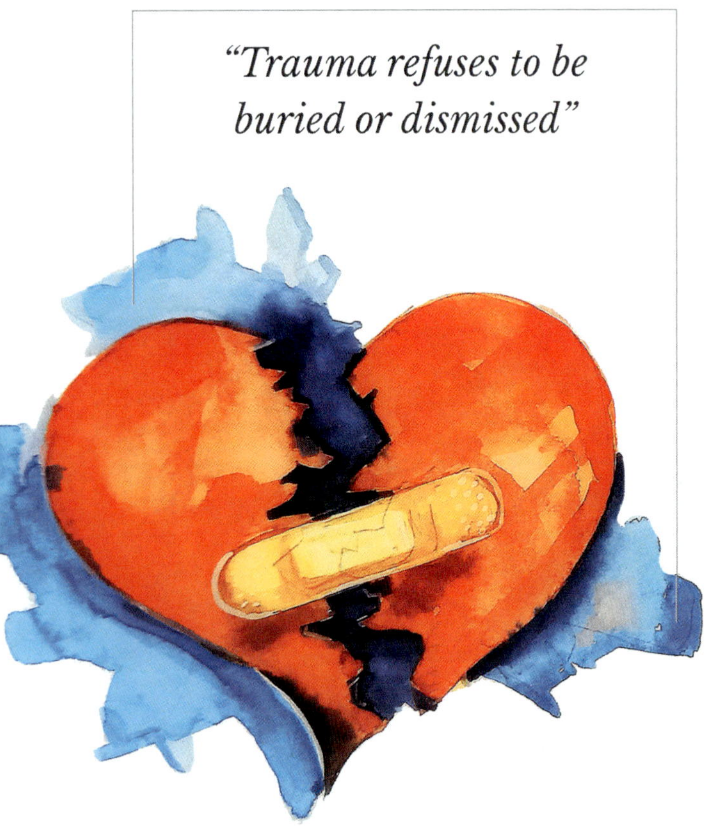

Unhealed trauma will appear in diverse ways over the course of your lifetime. It can present as psychological distress symptoms such as anxiety, worry, fear, depression or addictions.

The more dreadful and monstrous the trauma, the more intense and pervasive the symptoms. Many people vacillate between numbing the symptoms and reliving the disturbing event.

These wounds will last until they are healed. Some people keep them for a lifetime.

The Nature of Wounds
The Open Wound

Most of us grazed our knees in childhood. Some of us have had more serious injuries as we grew older. Open wounds are raw, tender and sore. If they are unhealed, they will remain this way.

Every time you are triggered by someone touching your open physical wounds - you will recoil in pain. Your unhealed emotional wounds, even if suffered a long time ago, will respond in a similar way and the trauma happens all over again, i.e. re-traumatisation. This aspect is often the cause of many conflicts in relationships. Triggering occurs mainly through your five senses- sight (eg. watching a child cry), smell (eg. of blood or fire), touch (eg. being grasped or inappropriately touched), sound (eg. raised voices or gunshots) or taste (eg. salty saliva).

Once triggered, the rawness of your wound opens up and your reaction will be out of proportion to the current event. This means that the old torment is happening all over again due to unhealed wounds.

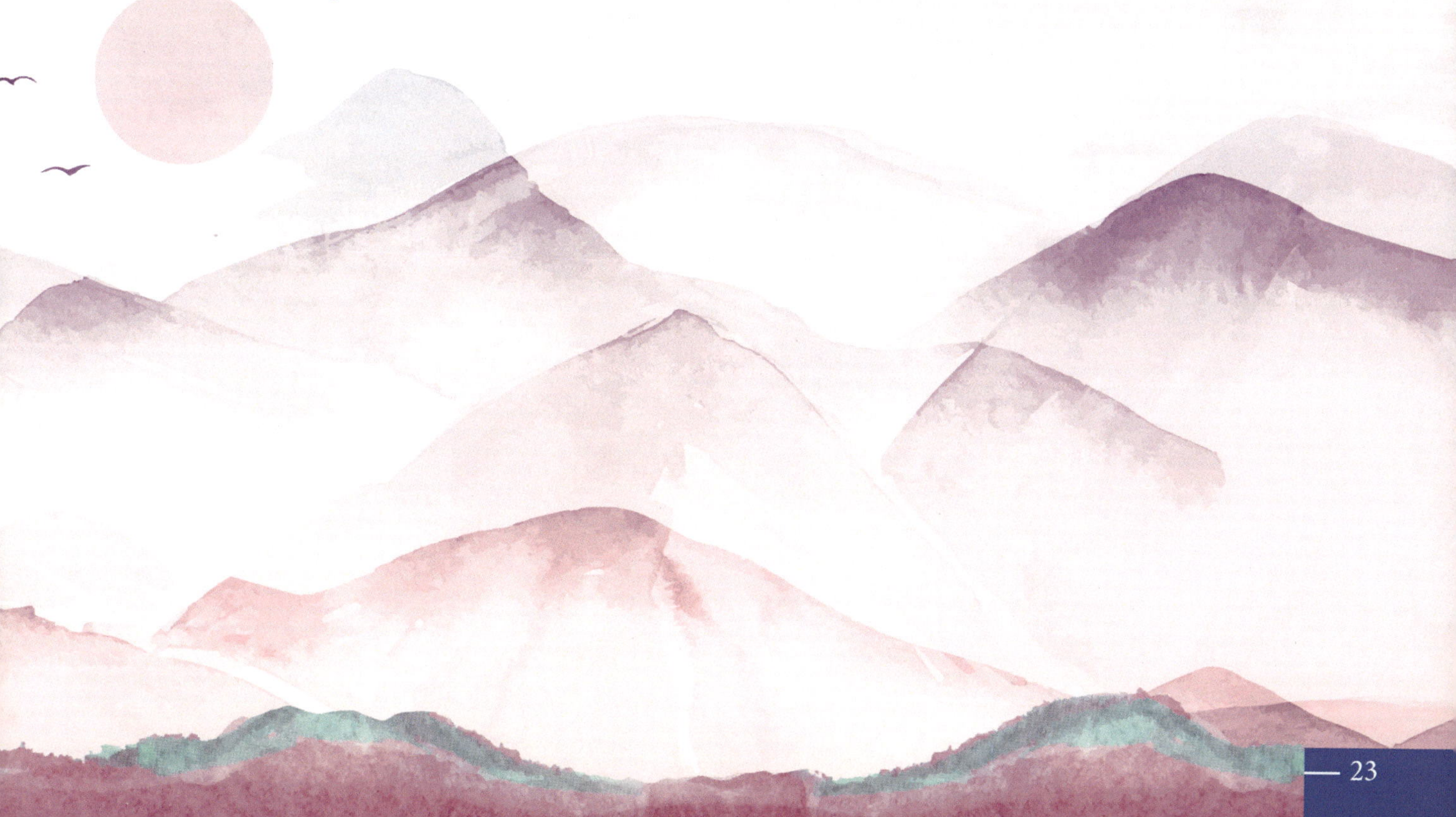

The Scar

Over time wounds can turn into scars. My patients have called their scars battle wounds and gone to great lengths to disguise their appearance. The holding onto psychological scars can sculpt lives and last for generations eg. unhealed scars of war.

Scar tissue has certain distinct features.

◆ Scars become very hard over time. This is true in people who have suffered emotional trauma. Hardness is protective, but it can become the place of bitterness and resentment.

◆ Scars can become inflexible and rigid. Many patients attempt to control their environment and the people in it. This is often to their detriment, because the control proves to be illusive when new trauma arrives at their doorstep.

◆ Scars constrict. Over time scars will contract, stunt or even stop growth. no longer seen as a place of opportunity, purpose and adventure, but one of fear and anxiety.

◆ Scars become callous and lose sensation. Scar tissue has no nerve endings and this leads to numbness, apathy and indifference. Many people carrying trauma become numb to everyday life and the gift of healing.

Let's dig deeper into understanding trauma...

The Tree Diaries

A hundred-year-old botanical garden lies at the heart of Durban. The garden is a leafy space where locals gather for leisurely walks, picnics and celebratory photo shoots. It is not uncommon to find a few tree stumps in the garden. These tree stumps have a number of circular growth rings on the surface - which show every single year the tree has been in existence. These growth rings tell us the life story of the tree. It's a historical record and a cryptic diary.

The width, thickness and colour of each growth ring reveal the details of what the tree experienced in a particular year.

A single circle can show a bleak drought. Another circle will reveal that the tree was struck by lightning. Other circles could expose healthy years of growth, forest fires, avalanches, earthquakes, or a year of disease. It is a library of information - a natural archive and a precise record.

We too are like trees and have circles of our own traumas. An imprint of unresolved trauma from every year exists. Just like a tree keeps records, every hurt experienced, harsh word spoken, every rejection and trace of fear has been recorded. Every time we are abandoned, overwhelmed or threatened, the bad experience is stored. Current life events eg. a global pandemic, earthquake or personal crisis can have the effect of ripping the bark off the tree. Then the layers of hurt underneath come into sight. For some, it can be a lifetime of unhealed bruises.

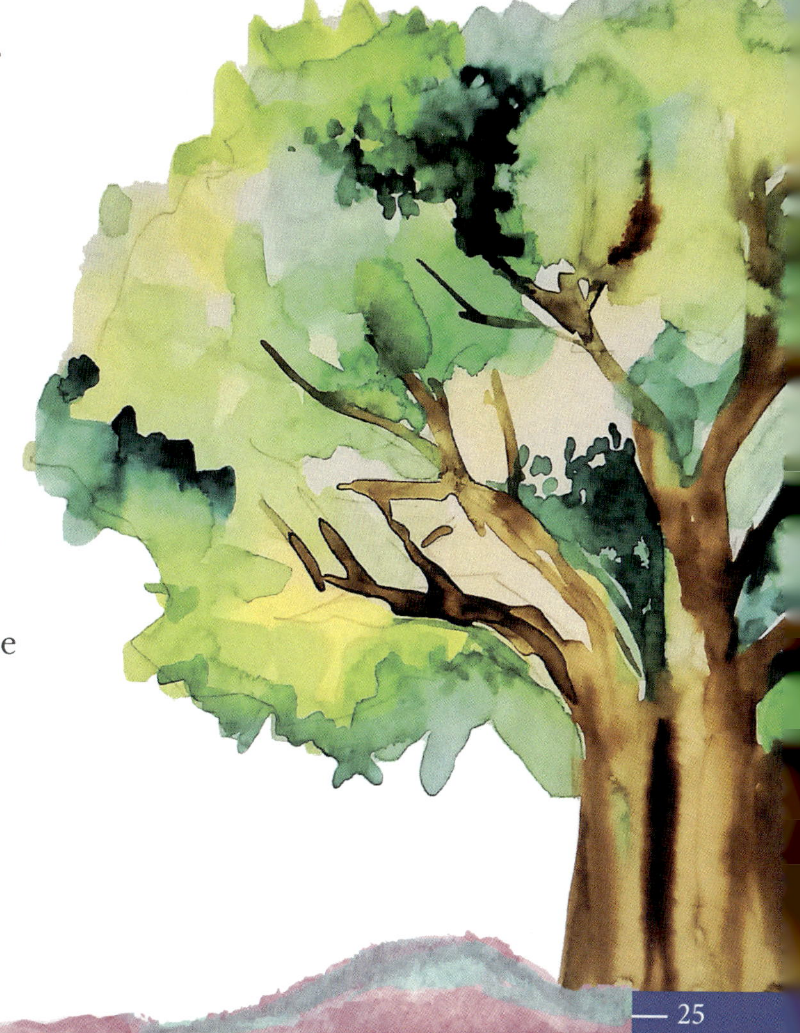

Chapter Two

What are these hurts that can be found in the rings of your tree of life?
Firstly, there are ancient wounds found in the first circle of your history - this is the trauma experienced in your mother's womb. If she was anxious, afraid or abandoned, those emotions can be transferred to you as an unborn child in the womb.
She could have had financial stress and no family support.These hurts can be embedded in the first or innermost circle, the cradle of the tree.

Secondly, there are innumerable scars that can emerge from childhood experiences. *I recall a patient, Maya, telling me about herself as a little girl, sitting on the porch in her prettiest dress, waiting for her father to visit.*

Maya's mother was his mistress. Her father had promised to bring her a gift and take her to play in the nearby park. Maya waited, looking down the road for a tall man to walk towards her.

He never arrived. As a psychologist, I know that the rejection by a father creates a wound that can last a lifetime. Little Maya proceeded to blame herself for his absence. She wondered if she was a naughty little girl, or maybe she was not pretty enough? That crucial day began her search for perfection. This scar was a stain on her life and it has eaten away at her soul, causing numerous problems in her marriage. Her childhood hurt did not go away. It was buried just beneath the bark of the tree and needed healing.

Some patients have dark tragic rings. This is a wicked imprint of someone older taking advantage of their vulnerable childhood and introducing them to the violation of sexual abuse. Years ago, I treated forty-year-old Liam.

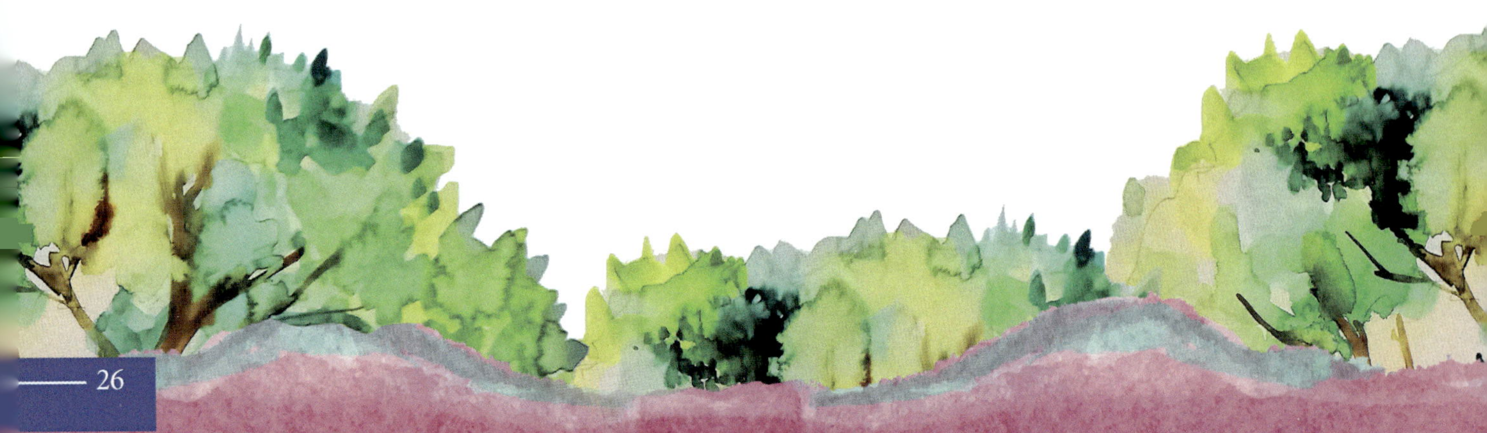

Chapter Two

As an innocent young boy, his uncle abused him sexually and this muddied the rest of his life. Liam was awaiting the birth of his own son when his life became undone. In hospital, he admitted that he had struggled with depression and cocaine addiction for most of his life. This was the beginning of his journey of healing and embracing fatherhood.

The scar of emotional neglect by parents and other caregivers is prevalent in most of my patients. Parents can be dismissive, neglectful or demeaning.

Many homes are tempestuous and display aggression in words and deeds. **I treated an astute lawyer named Nicole who was on the cutting edge in her field.** However, her relationships, both platonic and romantic, were erratic and unpredictable. Her temperament could change quickly from mild irritation to intense rage.

As we unpacked her history in therapy, we found that she buried herself in academics to avoid the violence between her parents. There were fights and loud arguments that could last into the early hours of the morning. These scars of a fearful child witnessing trauma were concealed for most of her life. Nicole could not understand that while she was successful in every area of her life, she could not sustain personal relationships.

Our work together focussed on breaking these patterns and healing the wounds of parental neglect. Each of us has our own rings of psychological pain.

It is a record written in our hearts and minds that is still alive but suppressed. Nothing just goes away. Nothing is erased. It affects how we view life. It also affects how we view ourselves and all relationships. My work as a psychotherapist is about looking past the hard exterior bark. It's about allowing people a sacred space in my office to take down their masks so that we may see what is underneath and begin the journey to wholeness.

Personal Reflection
The Rings of the Tree of your Life

If we look at a cross-section of your life, what stories of trauma and joy will the rings of your history tell us? What will we find under the protective bark of your tree of life?

Write a short paragraph outlining **your recent painful incidents and experiences.**
This could be abuse, unfair treatment, the death of a loved one, loss of a significant relationship, being a victim of violence or even hurtful words spoken to you or about you.

Thoughts:

Write about **your childhood memories (age 1-6 years old).** These are the inner rings of your tree. Record the painful and positive experiences.

Thoughts:

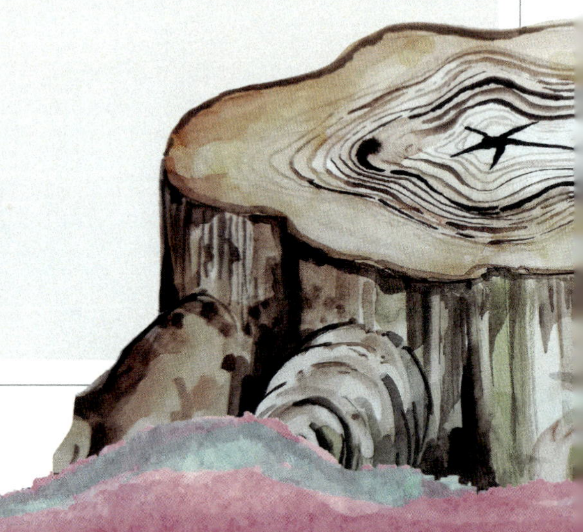

Personal Reflection
The Rings of the Tree of your Life

If we look at a cross-section of your life, what stories of trauma and joy will the rings of your history tell us? What will we find under the protective bark of your tree of life?

There are rings dedicated to **our school and teenage years.** Write down any painful or positive life shaping memories from that period of life.

Thoughts:

Adulthood is a time of transitions - studying, working, relationships, parenting and more. Write down five experiences that have shaped your journey as an adult.

Thoughts:

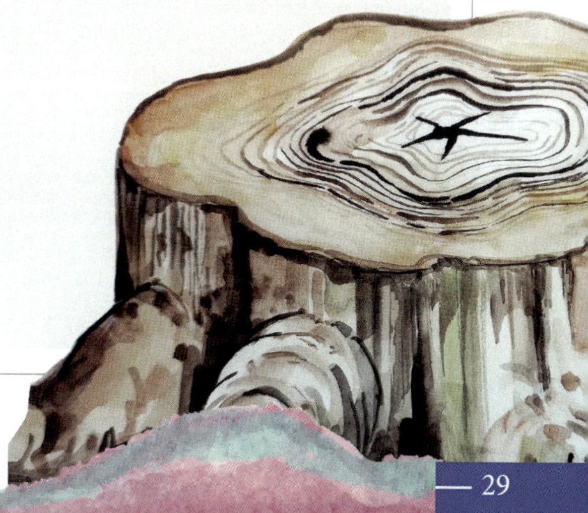

Personal Reflection

Personal Reflection

PART I

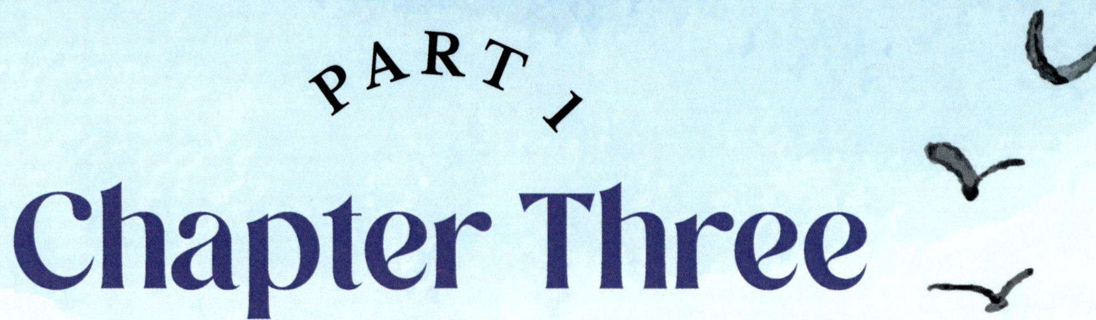

Chapter Three

Divine Architecture

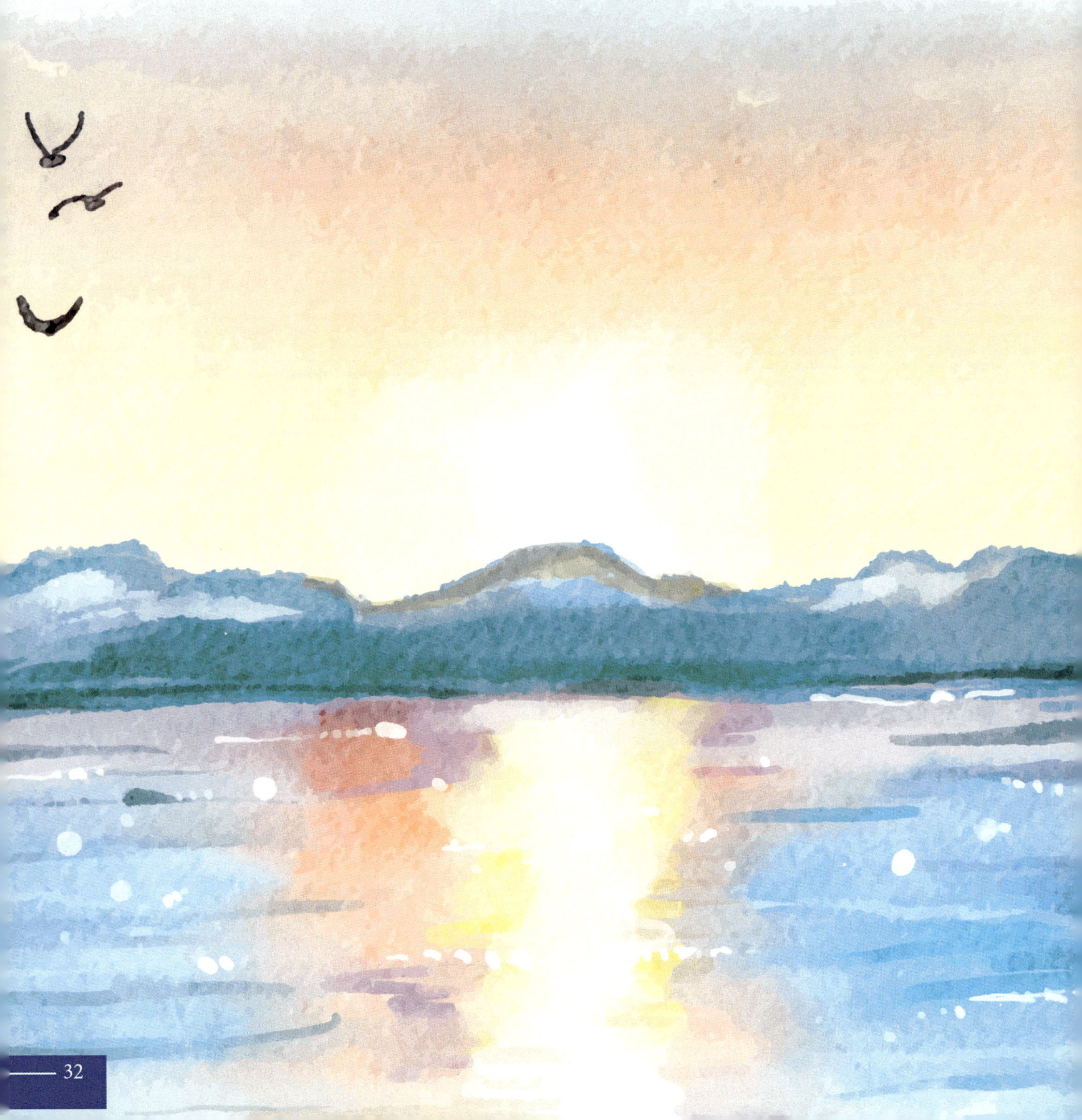

The Allure of Istanbul

Istanbul in Turkey is a captivating city that is spread across two continents. It is an exotic location where East meets West. I was on a yacht sailing down the Bosporus Strait, which runs through the city and connects the Black Sea and the Sea of Marmara. The architectural wonders of empires past create a skyline that is ancient and alluring.

While sipping on a Turkish coffee, I watched Byzantine churches, Ottoman mansions, pavilions, ornate minarets and stately towers with intricate designs embrace the shoreline. As my senses delighted in this design feast, I was reminded that all humanly crafted beauty could not compare to the architecture that is us - **you and I.**

We are an elegantly crafted balance of Spirit, Soul and Body.
Each part separate yet able to flow together.
Connected but not interchangeable.
Majestic in every way imaginable.
A distinct Divine Architecture.

When you understand the intimate construction and dynamic workings of your composition, a new window of insight about healing opens to you. God created you with three distinct parts- a body, a soul and a spirit. This is penned in First Thessalonians, Chapter 5, verse 23: 'Now may the God of peace Himself sanctify you completely; and may your whole spirit, soul, and body be preserved blameless at the coming of our Lord Jesus Christ'. God intentionally created you this way. Healing and Wholeness begins in your spirit and your soul and body bathe in its benefits.

Let us learn more about each part.

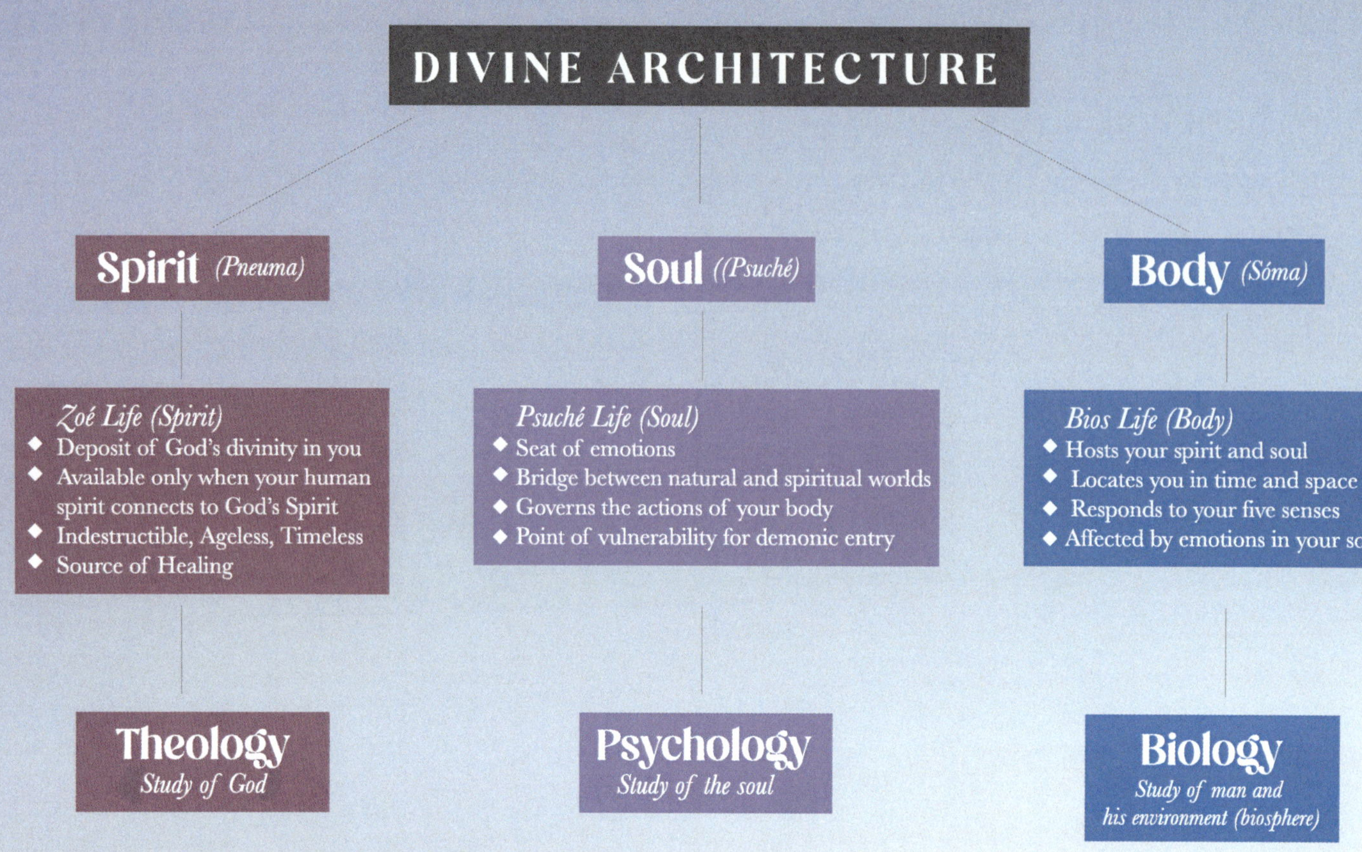

A Divine Framework: Spirit and Soul

God constructed your spirit and soul to function in tandem.

- They are mirrors of each other because God designed your soul to live under the rulership of your spirit.
- Your spirit has a mind and your soul has a mind.
- Your spirit has a will and your soul has a will.
- Your spirit has a heart and your soul has a heart.
- The Divine order is your spirit (connected to the Spirit of God) ruling over your soul and your soul ruling over your body.

Understanding the Spirit of God and the Human Spirit

The Spirit of God is a life-giving Spirit. When the first man, Adam, received an impartation of Spirit from God, he received more than the ability to breathe. He received an awareness of the presence of God and a connection to his Creator. This spirit which came out of the very person of God is indestructible and in death moves seamlessly from this world back to God. We too have been given this exact divine deposit from God.

The Spirit of God is an endowment of His divine nature into you. It is ageless and timeless. If the spirit of God could be envisioned as a vast ocean - then each one of us receives a bucket of that ocean into our beings. This 'bucket of ocean' has all the elements of the ocean, but, as you are aware, you cannot sail a ship in a bucket.

Let's delve deeper and understand the soul when disconnected from the Spirit of God.

SPIRIT & SOUL (EACH HAS THREE DIMENSIONS)

◆ *Mind:* organ of perception to view current reality, challenges and certainties.

◆ *Will:* Source of intelligence and place of decision- making. The will is the intelligence used to put together available resources.

◆ *Heart:* Control room of all motivation and determines your actions. Seat of emotional life - every human decision is based on emotion and justified by reason.

SPIRIT (MIND)

01 Sees everything from an eternal, timeless point of view.

02 Embraces God as Father and self as His Son (child of God). Relies on the Father for all resources and security.

03 Relies on God's wisdom and understanding to inform reality.

04 Revelation resets the mind of the spirit.

SOUL (MIND)

01 Sees everything from an earthly point of view.

02 Sees self as the source of all provision and protection. Has no father and is a spiritual orphan.

03 Relies on the five senses to understanad reality.

04 Information resets the mind of the soul.

SPIRIT (WILL)

01 Powered by the Spirit of God.

02 Puts into action the gifts of the spirit, eg. Faith, Hope and Love

03 Has a clear Godly vision for life. Sees God as the architect of one's destiny.

04 Pursues only what God wants for life. Operates from a place of spiritual rest.

05 Relies on heavenly economies for life and trusts God for all provision and protection.

SOUL (WILL)

01 Powered by Self.

02 Lives a life of control, threats and manipulation.

03 Has own vision for life. Sees self as the architect of one's destiny.

04 Drives own destiny by own determination and stamina. Operates in constant fatigue and exhaustion.

05 Sees self as the source of all provision and protection. Always feels vulnerable.

SPIRIT (HEART)

01 Driven by perfect love which casts out all fear.

02 God's perfect love is an anchor for life.

SOUL (HEART)

01 Driven by fear and anxiety.

02 There is no reliable anchor for life.

Can a Believer have a demon?

No evil spirit has access or entrance into the sacred, inner sanctum of your spirit being. They cannot live where the Holy Spirit lives but they can live where they are given access.

A human being, even a believer in Christ, can unwittingly give access to a demon through their soul. An evil spirit cannot dwell where the Spirit of God dwells, in your spirit, but it can dwell in your soul. Your emotions live in your soul and the capture of your emotions is where evil spirits are able to achieve control-which in turn allows them to inhabit the soul. When they do, you do have fully active demonic capabilities functioning in your soul, manifesting in human behaviour, in the human body.

> *"I think it is clergy malpractice to look at people who are trapped in the schemes of the devil and to tell them it is their fault."*
> ~ Dr Sam Soleyn

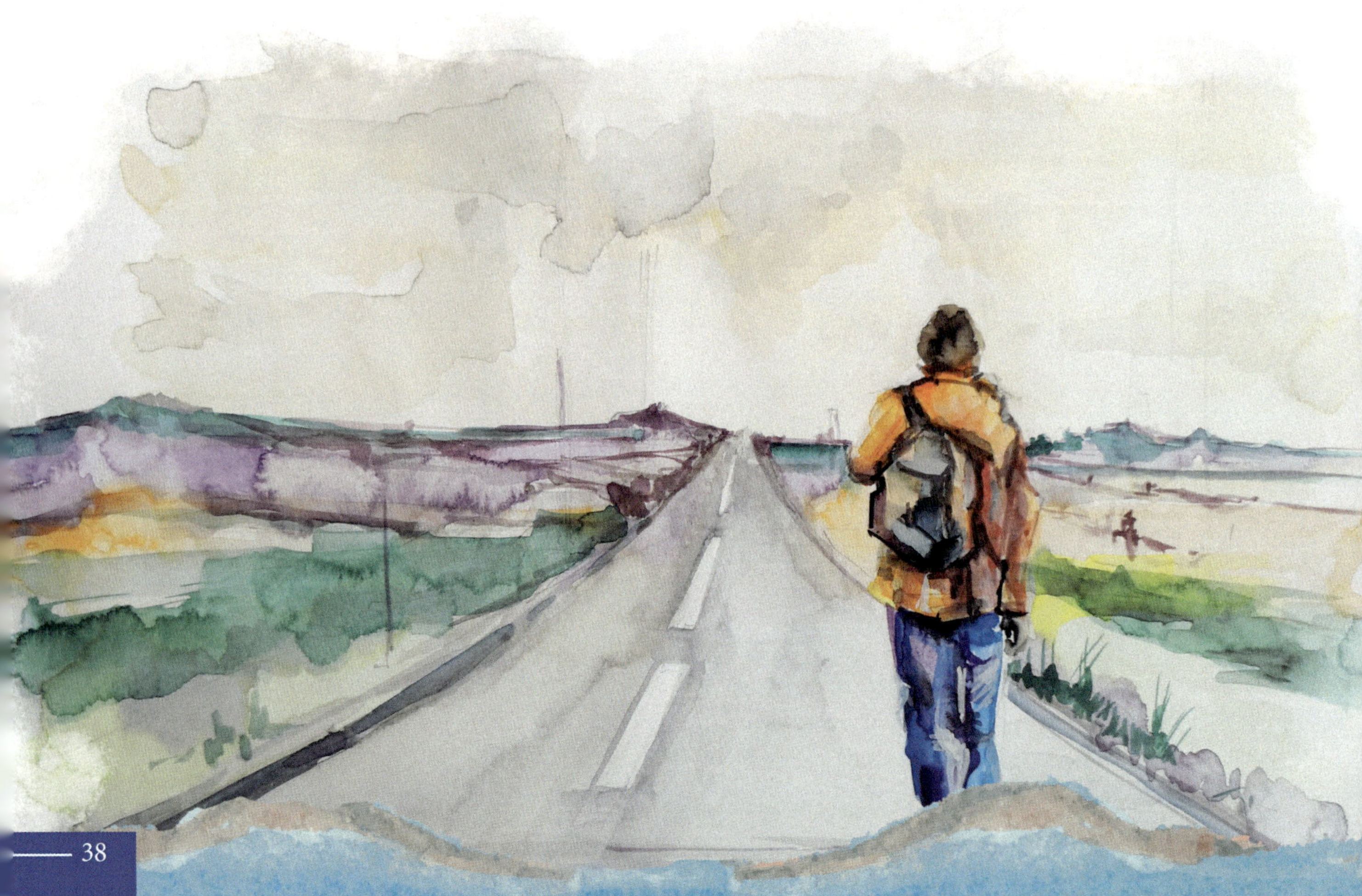

Understanding the Human Body

'My body is screaming', she said. Naledi is an entrepreneur who excels as a chiropractor, fitness coach and mother of three small children. However, she is trapped in an emotionally abusive marriage. The result has been her having a series of illnesses over the past years- one medical crisis after the next. As soon as Naledi's migraines improved, ulcers appeared. Once treated, she was diagnosed with a spinal disc inflammation. It has been an unending cycle. Emotional stress has wreaked havoc with her body.

More on the body...

◆ Our bodies were formed from the dust of the earth!

◆ The life that God placed in the body is called bios and the study of this life is biology.

◆ The body locates us in time and space and responds acutely to our five senses.

◆ Whatever we see, hear, touch, taste and smell has the effect of invoking an emotional response that is related to historical trauma- a reaction that can even take us back to an early childhood memory. This memory can be positive or negative and can impact the actions we take in the present moment.

◆ The body responds to the emotions in the soul and can become the source of many physical symptoms of illness.

◆ Psychosomatic illness is the link between your body and your emotions. Under stress and trauma, the first challenges are often experienced in the body, eg. insomnia, pain, fatigue, headaches or loss of appetite.

◆ Emotions that accompany these symptoms often include low mood, anxiety, fear and suicidal thoughts.

◆ Many people focus on healing the body and neglect the internal environment of the soul and spirit.

Personal Reflection

Understanding Anxiety and Fear Persistent anxiety is draining and fear causes us to become stuck. These two emotions affect different dimensions of your life. Below is a list of potential areas that may be impacted by these emotions.

Identify any area where anxiety or fear is a problem and write down a few notes detailing how these emotions are keeping you restricted in that aspect of life.

- Relationships
- Health
- Work
- Spiritual life
- Finances
- Family

Personal Reflection

Personal Reflection

PART 1

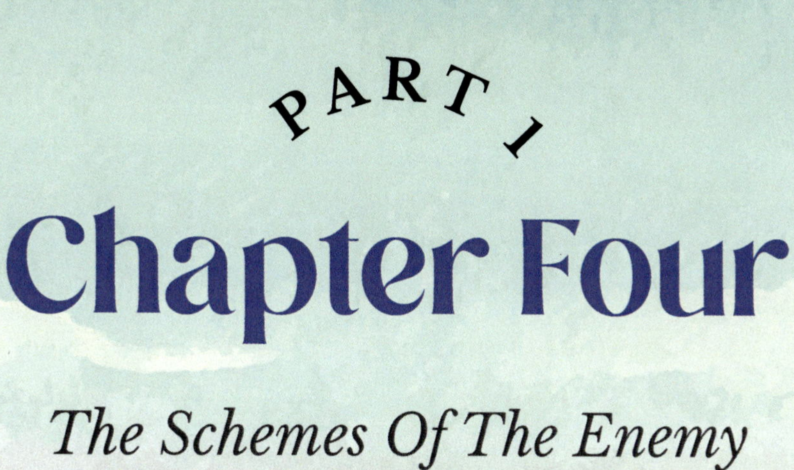

Chapter Four

The Schemes Of The Enemy

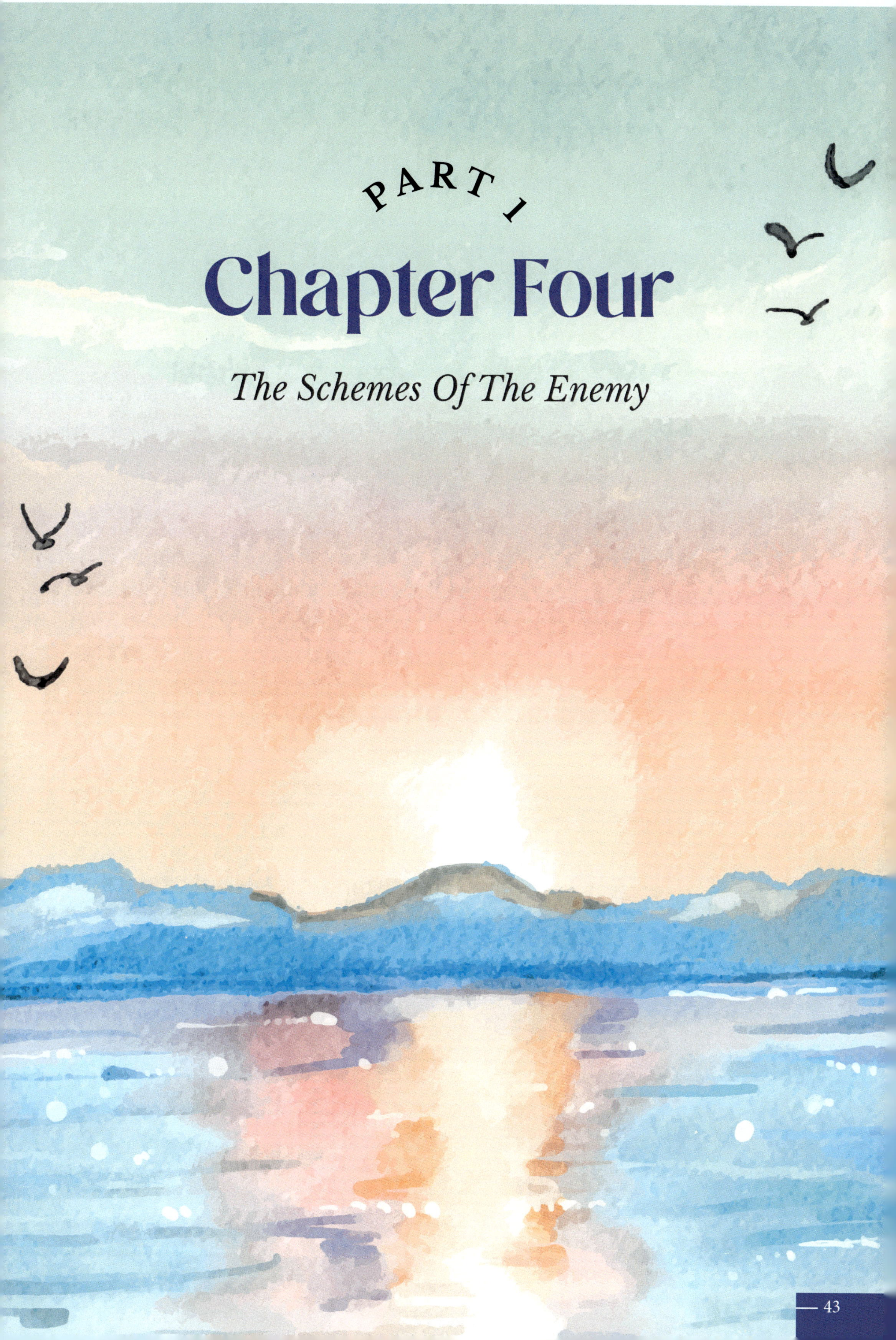

Chapter Four

What About Amelia?

Amelia was twenty-five years old. During her high school years she had a stellar academic record, was sporty and worked as a part-time model. However, as time progressed she entered a series of abusive romantic relationships that caused her to gradually become clinically depressed. In desperation, her family took her to priests, shamans and fortune tellers. Her depression became acute and she was consumed with suicidal feelings.

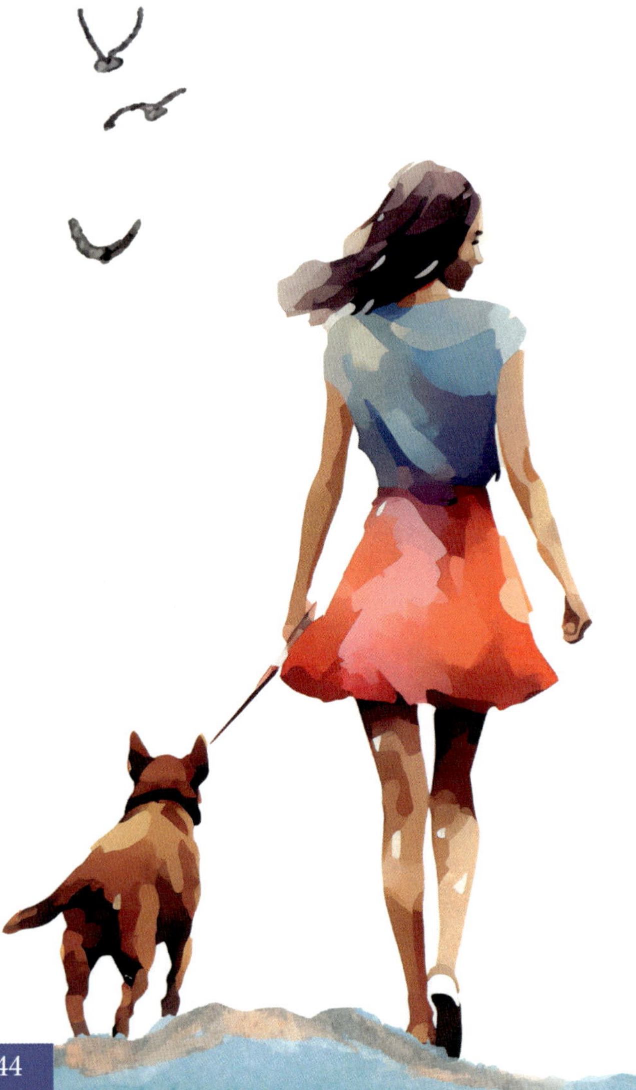

Amelia also began to hear voices that urged her to kill herself.

I first met Amelia in a psychiatric ward. Her hair was matted and her clothing mismatched. Amelia's face was distressed and she said: 'The voices are telling me not to listen to you and they want me to run out of this room'. She repeatedly told me that she just wanted to die. However, Amelia began to improve on her medication and Electroconvulsive Therapy (ECT). This is a treatment procedure that involves small electric currents passing through the brain and has been effective in preventing suicide in certain patients.

Unfortunately Amelia and I only saw each other when she was admitted to hospital. This began happening every two months and then more frequently. Her suicidal thoughts grew more intense. In sessions she now growled and barked at me. She told me that the voices grew louder in my presence. Her psychiatrist and I were reaching the end of our efforts. We admitted our limitations and knew that we were facing a situation that was beyond the scope of our clinical and diagnostic training.

What About Amelia? Continued

One day, another psychiatrist noticed Amelia growling and snarling in the hospital corridor.

'What force was that?' she wondered.
'This case is for a priest, not a therapist', she insisted.
We agreed with her and took the bold step of offering to bring in a pastor, who was proficient in dealing with such cases, to administer his methods of care to her. The family approved. The pastor intervened with prayer to identify and remove demonic spirits that plagued Amelia. She started to improve after a single intervention. However, on discharge from hospital she continued visiting tribal healers, mediums and spiritualists whom she had consulted earlier. The voices returned more viciously than before.

Amelia refused any further therapy sessions and was only willing to take her medication. The last time I spoke to her was at her hospital bedside. Her breakfast had been brought to her and a butter knife lay on the plate. She spent time staring at the knife and then staring at me - back and forth. I had a strong sense that she wanted to harm me. I stepped back. She thanked me for trying to help her and said goodbye to me.

A few months later Amelia committed suicide from a medication overdose. All her treating doctors were deeply saddened. What was the force that had taken over her mind and eventually caused her to kill herself? What growled at me and threatened to attack me? Was it a force of prime evil? I believe that it was and that her soul was inhabited by it. In clinical practice, I have seen evil overrun patient's lives - in overt and covert ways. It is time to understand and heal people entrapped by the schemes of the enemy.

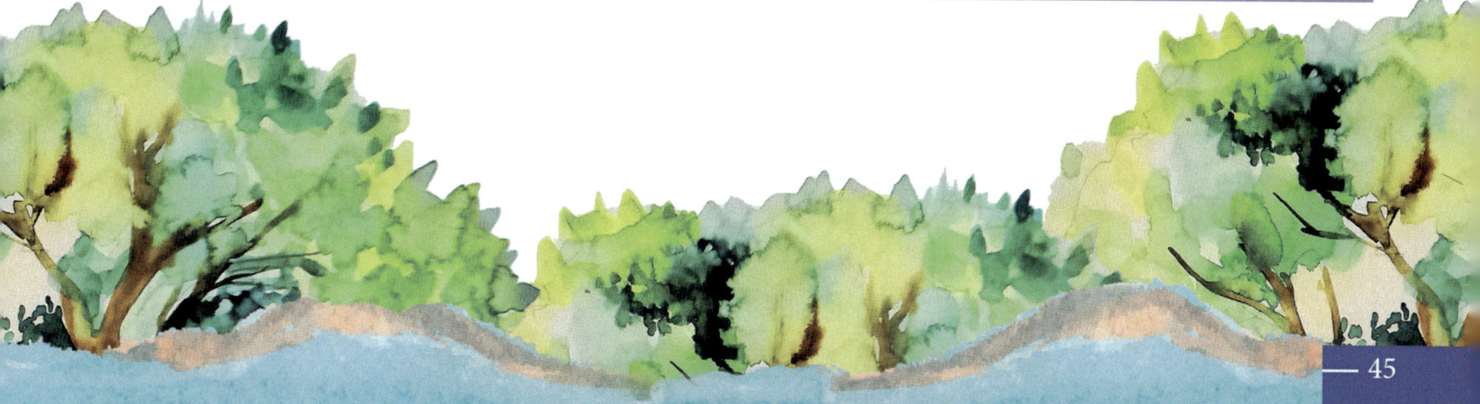

Who is the Enemy?

"Put on the full armour of God so that you can take your stand against the devil's schemes. For our struggle is not against flesh and blood, but against the rulers, against the authorities, against the powers of this dark world and against the spiritual forces of evil in the heavenly realms". **(Ephesians 6: 11-12)**

The biblical description of the devil or Satan is vastly different from the one seen in popular culture and social media.

◆ In the scriptures he is NOT the animated cartoon character who is dressed in long red tights with horns, a tail and a pitchfork.

◆ Satan is a formidable adversary who has been profiling your weaknesses and traumas for generations.

◆ He uses deception, stratagems and trickery to exploit every weakness in your soul.

◆ Satan's intent is to craft an alternative to God. This substitute is driven by your fears. However, if your life is under the lordship of the Spirit of God, these schemes are ineffective and have little ability to impact you.

The Bible calls the devil your enemy and labels him as 'the deceiver of the whole world'. He is also called the accuser (Revelation 12:9-10), 'the ruler of this world' (John 12:31), and 'the god of this age' (2 Corinthians 4:4). Satan is our 'adversary who prowls around like a roaring lion, seeking someone to devour' (1 Peter 5:8).

He is also referred to as 'the prince of the power of the air, the spirit that is now at work in the sons of disobedience' (Ephesians 2:2). In the book of John (10:10) we are warned that the thief comes to steal, kill and destroy. Overall, Satan is an evil genius, a mastermind who seeks to bring chaos, confusion and destruction to you. Satan and other fallen angels have an extensive understanding of the human soul and are able to motivate other human beings to act against you. Fear is often the driving emotion that causes others to oppose you, without any just cause.

Who is the Enemy?

Where does Satan come from?

Before God created the earth, He brought into existence heavenly realms of authority and order.

- As part of this divine design, a multitude of angels were created as ministering servants to God and humans.
- These angels are spirits, but have no influence on the human spirit, which is under the domain of God's Spirit.
- Angels were not created as children of God - only we humans have that right and privilege.
- Angels have rankings, the highest of which is an archangel. Michael and Gabriel are named in scripture as archangels.
  Satan was also an archangel who was the head of praise and worship to God. His original name, Lucifer, means 'light-bearer'.
- Satan and one-third of the angels rebelled against God's choice of humans as His heirs. Only humans have the capacity to carry God's spiritual image and likeness.
- The fallen angels warred against God and questioned
- His authority and the ordering of creation. All of those were expelled from the heavenly realm of God's throne (Luke 10:18).
- Since the fall of Adam, they have been roaming the earth bringing destruction and chaos to human lives by entrapping the souls of people.

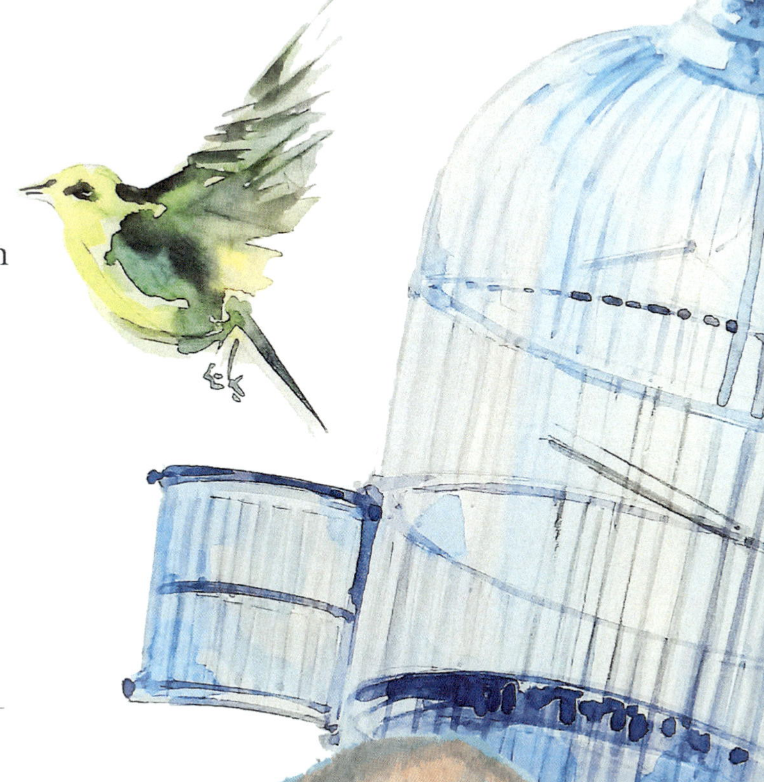

Rhea's Senses

The competence of angels is to serve your soul or to exploit it. My patient Rhea told me that every time she watches a movie where an actor is crying, she gets emotional and remembers the many months she spent in tears on her bedroom floor. She expressed that she was flooded by memories of helplessness and hopelessness. This makes her forget all the gains she has made in therapy. In this instance the enemy used her senses of sight and sound to evoke painful memories that brought forth intense emotions. This eventually drove Rhea to suicidal thoughts.

The soul is the greatest point of vulnerability for a demonic attack. Angels understand your soul even better than you do.

Behind Enemy Lines

It is crucial to remember that Satan is strategic, sophisticated and precise. He operates in packs or prides in the same way as predators like wolves, lions and hyenas do. Packs vary in their composition. Whenever one demon gains access, it moves to consolidate control of the person by inviting others. There are several of these packs, and some are as different from the other packs as lions are different from wolves or dogs. Their opportunities are based in the scope of the trauma the host experiences. A pack led by the spirit of rejection will strengthen its position by inviting the spirits of abandonment, unworthiness, irrelevance, unimportance and sickness. If the pack is led by fear it will draw in the spirits of anxiety, worry, torment, shame and depression. If a pack is led by the spirit of humiliation, the pack will fortify its position with the spirits of shame, adultery, fornication, pornography and guilt. The gift of discerning between spirits is key to identifying the different packs - so that they may be cast out. As a child of God this gift is freely available to you when you ask the Lord to show you what is hidden in your soul.

Chapter Four

Tactical Advantages

Demonic attacks are well thought out plans, stratagems and schemes in the battleground of the human soul. Your enemy has two distinct tactical advantages over you: being invisible and having a longer life span. As humans, we are limited by time and space and will be outmatched by an invisible enemy. When considering the longer life span, remember that Satan was present in the Garden of Eden. He has been around for millennia and this gives him the distinct advantage of observing the pattern of each of our human lives. He compiles information about all our consistencies and inconsistencies from generation to generation. Imagine a file with your name on it with all your generational information - including people you have never known or met. Satan formulates a scheme to attack you in your soul through the abuse of your emotions. He is persistent and unrelenting in his attempts to prevent you from taking your rightful position as an heir of God and fulfilling the divine purpose for which you were created.

Life in the Spirit

The only way to overcome the onslaught of your enemy is to allow the Spirit of God to act on your behalf. The enemy knows that if he can control the emotions in your soul, he can bring you to a state of inner turmoil. In crisis your soul will want to disconnect from your spirit. That's his primary modus operandi. Many people in emotional crisis say things like 'Where is God?' or 'God has forsaken me'. In this state, your soul has separated from your spirit. At this point, your body will also become affected by the tumult in your soul. Emotions like depression and anxiety will often cause sleep disturbances, fatigue, pain and even neurological symptoms. Satan uses emotional trauma to entrap you and take over your mind and will. In summary, if your enemy can control your reactions to circumstances, he will control your decision-making. And that is his real power over you.

Setting the Captives Free

'My father is not demented, he is tormented'.
Ashton's 87-year-old Dad was curled up into a ball in his nursing home crib
bed. His life was slowing ebbing out of him. The room had the sulphuric smell
of gangrene. As Ashton took his father's hand to comfort him, a fierceness
manifested in his Dad. He tried to twist Ashton's hand, his face contorted and
he growled at him.

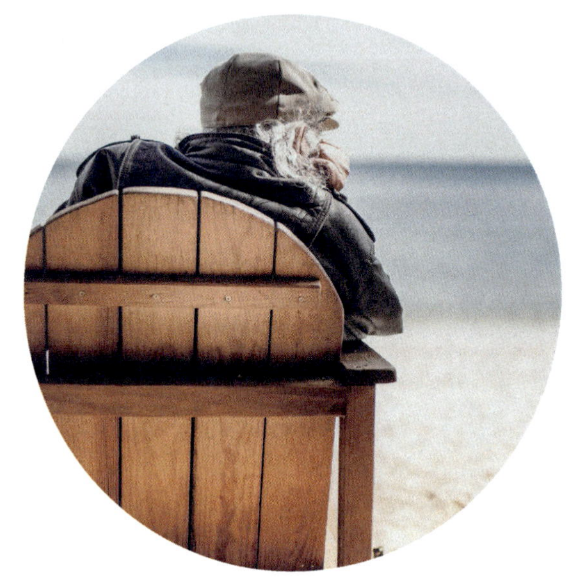

I have known Ashton for ten years and we
meet once a month for an introspective
healing conversation. He is forty years old,
a man of science who is discovering a path
with Jesus. We spoke about the aggressive
spirit that was haunting his father on his
deathbed - tormenting his mind and those
that had to watch his unbearable suffering.
*His father needed to be released from
evil and from this world back to God.*

This situation was beyond the boundaries of psychology so I encouraged
Ashton to pray for his father's last days. He chose The Lord's Prayer. On
his next visit, he held his father's hand and began to offer the prayer: 'My
Father who art in heaven, hallowed be thy name...'. His father was very
docile that day, but as Ashton prayed, he began to stir and respond to each
word with a sense of intrinsic connection and calm. Ashton improvised,
'deliver Dad from all evil', more than once. This prayer eased his Dad into
a gentle rest and the smell of gangrene vanished from the room. Two days
later he peacefully passed away.
Ashton's story shows us how the enemy inhabits the soul and torments the
mind, emotions and body of a person. There is trauma at every level and a
total entrapment. Only the Spirit of God breaks this bondage and frees the
person. *A gift of freedom available to all of us.*

Personal Reflection

Demonic Spirits

Your awareness and experience of demonic spirits changes over time. Your understanding may have been influenced by personal experience, observation of demonic activity in others, a spirit of discernment or religious teachings.

Write down your own journey of understanding and how you feel you have been impacted by demonic spirits.

Thoughts:

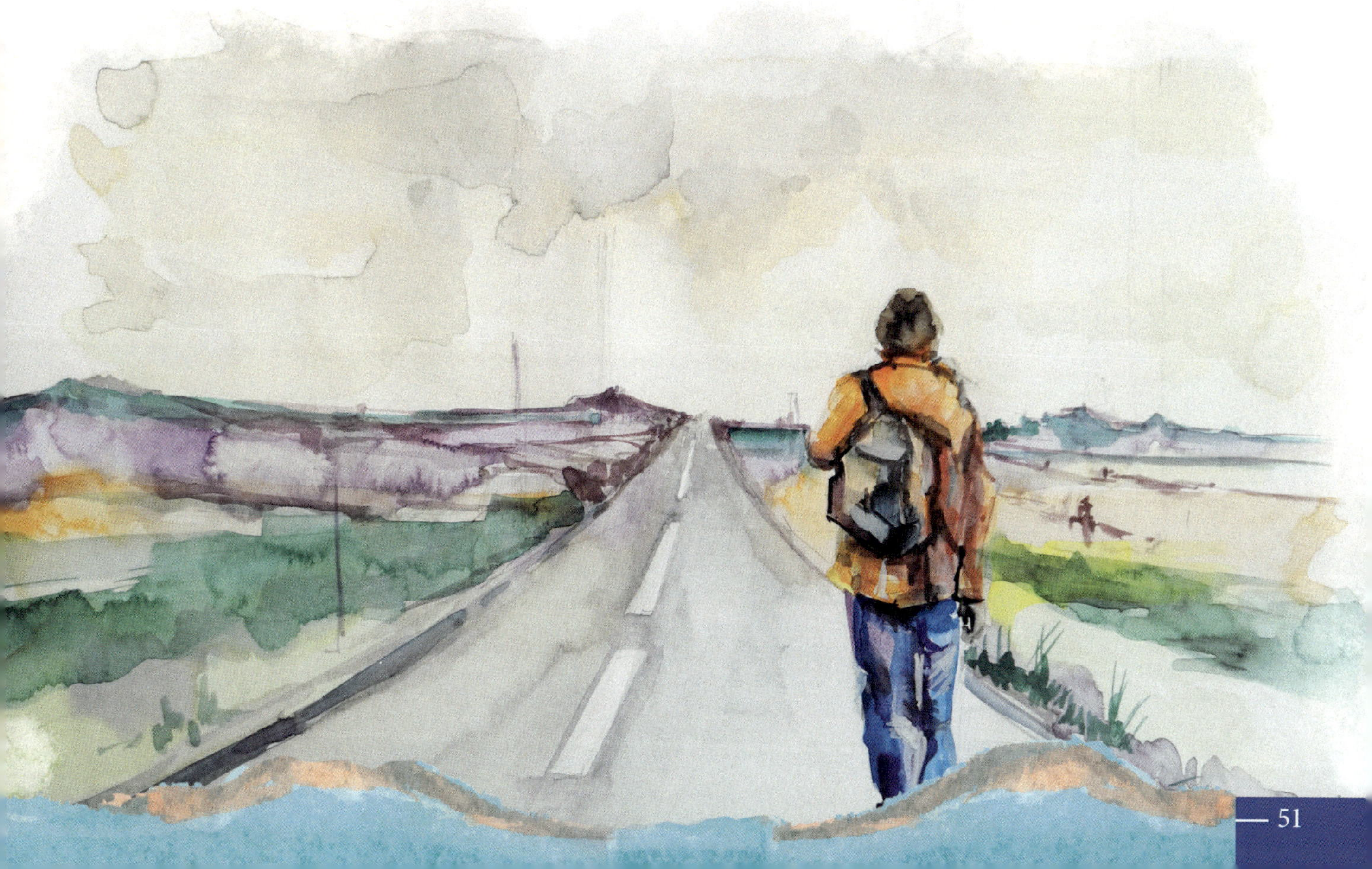

Personal Reflection

Personal Reflection

PART I

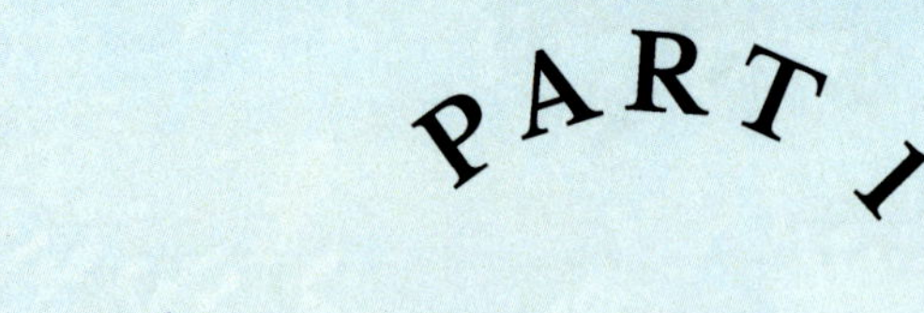

Chapter Five

Trauma In The Womb

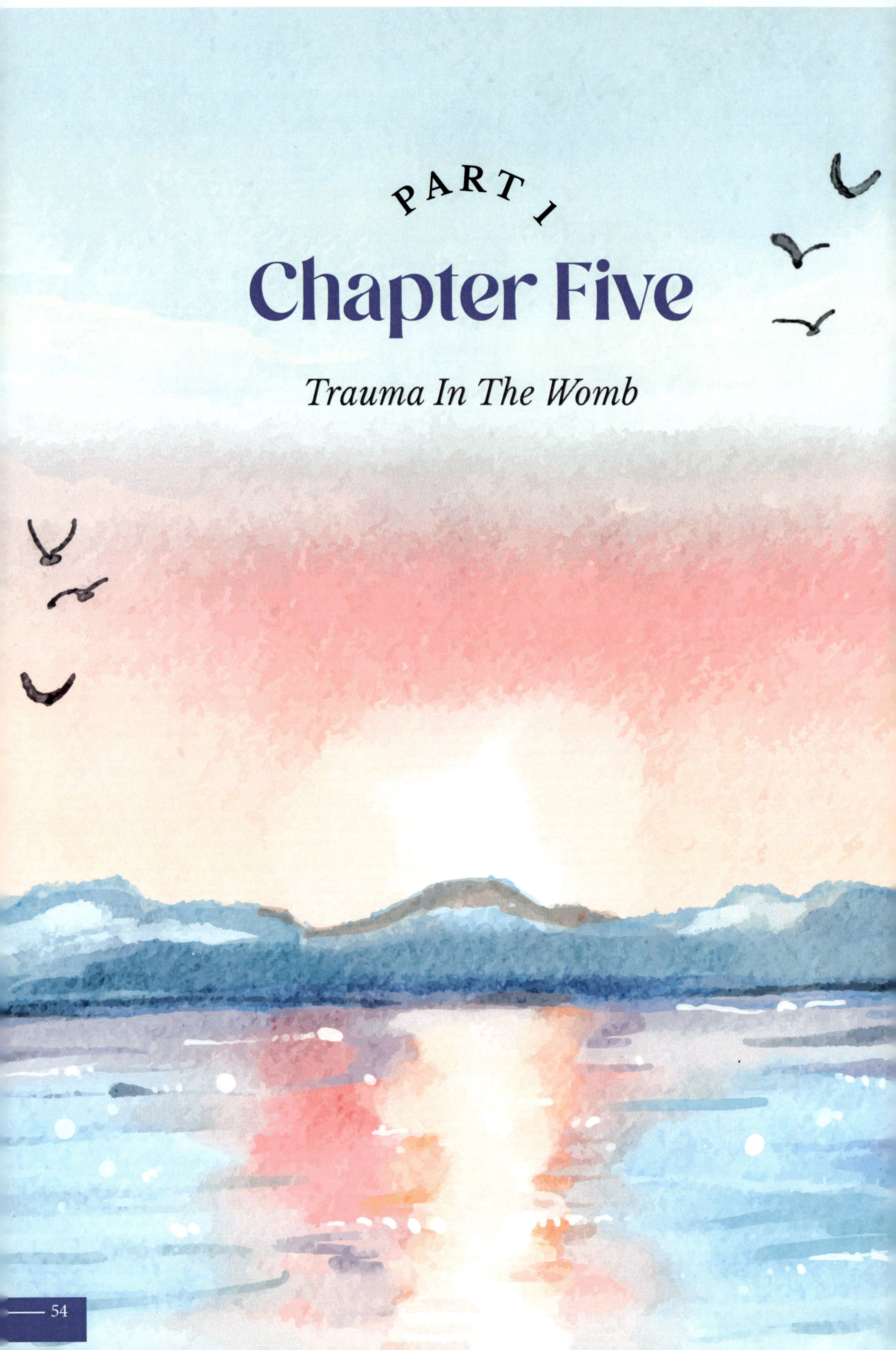

Echoes from the Womb

My experiences as a clinical psychologist have shown me that we are no tabula rasa. This is a Latin phrase that is often translated as 'blank slate'. 'It carries the notion that we are born empty, blank and devoid of a womb or ancestral history. This idea suggests that our identity is defined entirely by events after birth. I have found the opposite to be true. Experiences from conception and generational biographies shape our entire journey.

This chapter of the Workbook is an opportunity to delve deeper into your own in utero history and seek clues about the circumstances surrounding your development in the womb. You may be interested in learning the nature of your parents' relationship during the first forty weeks of your life. Let me share two stories from my clinical practice to give you deeper insight
- **those of Sadia and Jason.**

Chapter Five

Hidden in a Shoebox

Sadia was sitting at the edge of her hospital bed dangling her fluffy pink bedroom slippers. I noticed her long glossy hair. Her fearful gaze was surveying my face. Her right index finger pointed to her throat, indicating that she could not speak. She smiled weakly as I reached out my hand to shake hers - our first point of connection. It would take two days of anti-anxiety medication before she could communicate, albeit in whispering tones.

Thirty-two-year-old Sadia had lost all speech- a sinister silence had swallowed her words. It was not the first time. Sadia was born to a vulnerable 17-year-old schoolgirl who was not ready to be a mother. Her father was an anxious 21-year-old. Sadia's family rejected mother and child and asked her to hide her pregnancy and to give up the baby for adoption. A traditional marriage ensued on the insistence of her conservative parents.

Sadia's mother suffered immense fear, anxiety and shame. On her arrival into the world, baby Sadia became an object of public embarrassment.

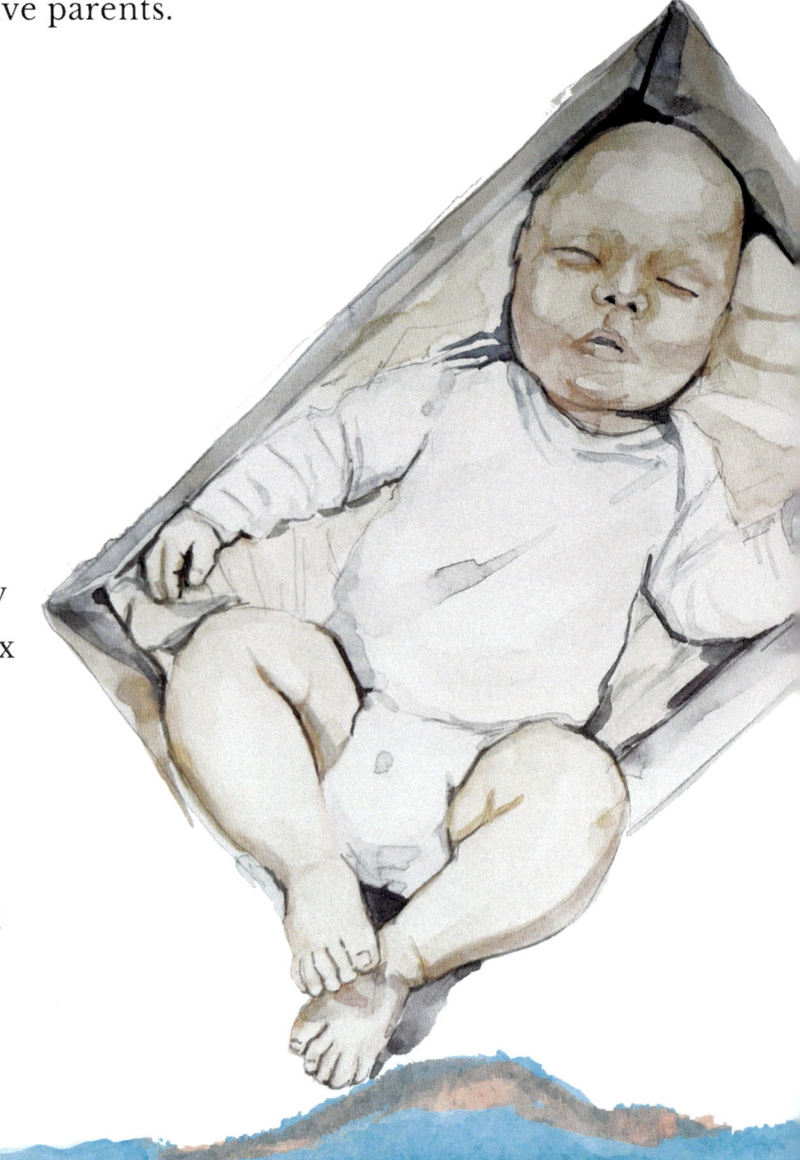

There was no celebration of her birth. There was no baby crib to call her own as she needed to be hidden away. Sadia was a tiny baby who fitted into a shoebox. This box was hidden behind the television cabinet when family visited. Instinctively, baby Sadia knew that she needed to be silent- no crying, no whimpering, no playful gurgling.

Hidden in a Shoebox Continued

The imprinted intrapsychic message was that her existence was irrelevant and that she was going to live voicelessly in the shadows. This was the beginning of her silence. In her early years at school she was labelled as having a learning disorder because she was unable to communicate freely. She also suffered physical hidings at the frustrated hands of her mother, who now had two more children. Sadia's rejection and sense of abandonment grew inside her and silence became her default setting.

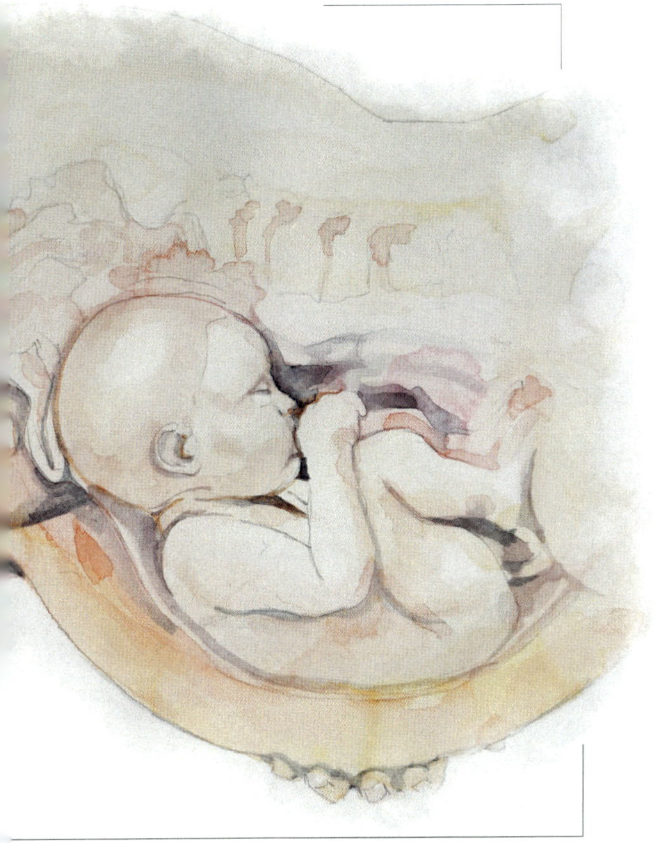

In high school, it was her father who encouraged her to complete her studies. Most of her relatives looked upon her with disdain and reinforced her sense of unworthiness. After school she entered an arranged marriage to a cruel man who physically abused her. She was forced to return home and felt am immense amount of shame. Years later, she remarried a kind and gentle man who had much patience with her. But Sadia struggled to share her thoughts and froze at any hint of criticism from him.

Now, 30 years later, the death of her father had once again collapsed her vocal cords. Grief had silenced her and threatened to engulf her entire being. She needed to find her words again, and never let them go. Over the next few months and years, Sadia healed from her losses and traumas and found her voice again. She recently graduated as a teacher.

The Primal Cry

Jason, a lanky 25-year-old graphic and mural artist, struggled with cannabis addiction, depression and debilitating anxiety. He had been admitted to the psychiatric ward following the breakup with his longtime girlfriend. This painful separation filled him with a sense of dread and unrelenting suicidal thoughts.

He was afraid to be outside the protective boundaries of the hospital. I asked him to sketch a picture to depict his inner turmoil, the parts of him that are unseen by the rest of the world. He drew a sad and disappearing face behind prison bars and wrote the number 25 in bold on the upper half of the page. He told me that this is him with a life sentenced to depression.

He felt trapped with no possibility of escape.

Jason's parents were undergoing a divorce and his mother Janet wanted to see me urgently. She was about to reveal a secret about his paternity that had been hidden for 25 years. She disclosed that Jason was a child born out of an affair with a colleague. At that point in time she lived in a small conservative rural town where gossip about her liaison became public knowledge.

Her pregnancy was filled with anxiety, terror and despair. Her husband agreed to adopt Jason and pretend that the child was his own biological offspring. His only condition was that Jason's true paternity never be revealed.

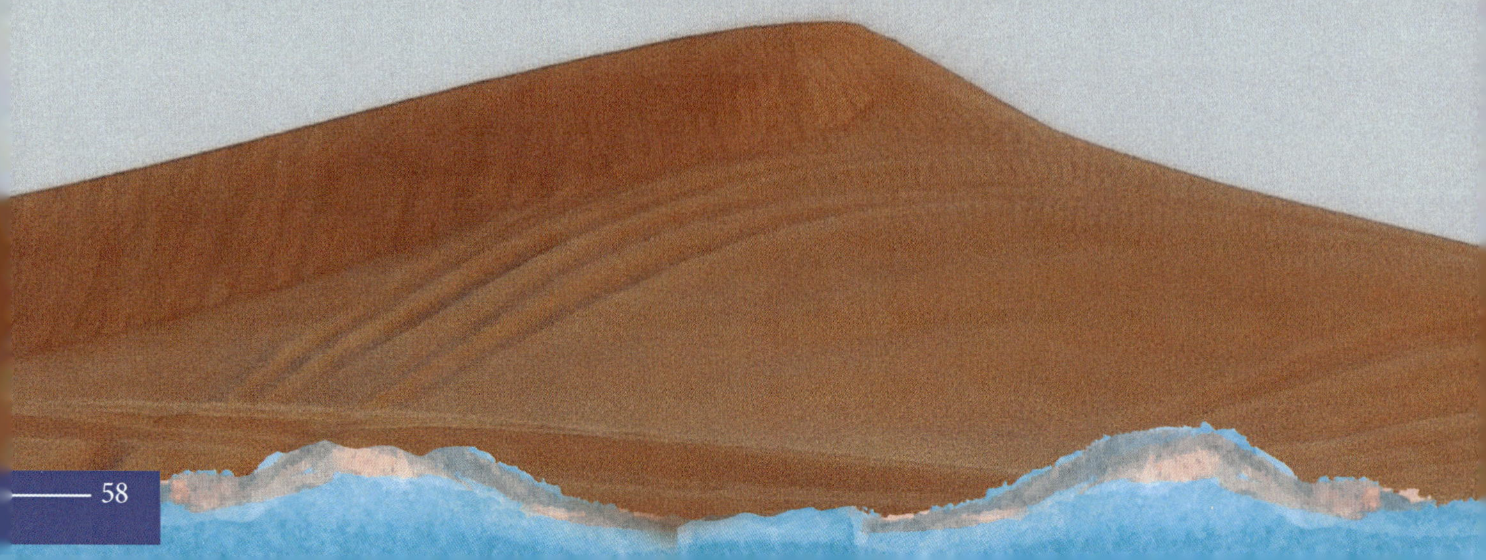

Chapter Five

The Primal Cry Continued

Now that they were getting a divorce, Janet felt she could emotionally unburden and free herself for the first time.

It was my daunting task to share this hidden information with a vulnerable Jason, as his parents were no longer on talking terms. He listened intently, tears welled in his light brown eyes, and then he broke out into a cry that came from a deep, almost ancestral place. It was a primal cry that expressed the depth of his loss and longing.

The next phase of his healing had opened up. In the weeks that followed, he felt freed from an emotional bondage that had stalked him all his life. He began the grief and forgiveness work in earnest - forgiving parents, others and himself for creating, maintaining and believing the lies about himself. *There is now a lightness in his pace and a peace that escapes human understanding. I had once again come face to face with womb trauma that daily shaped a young man's existence.*

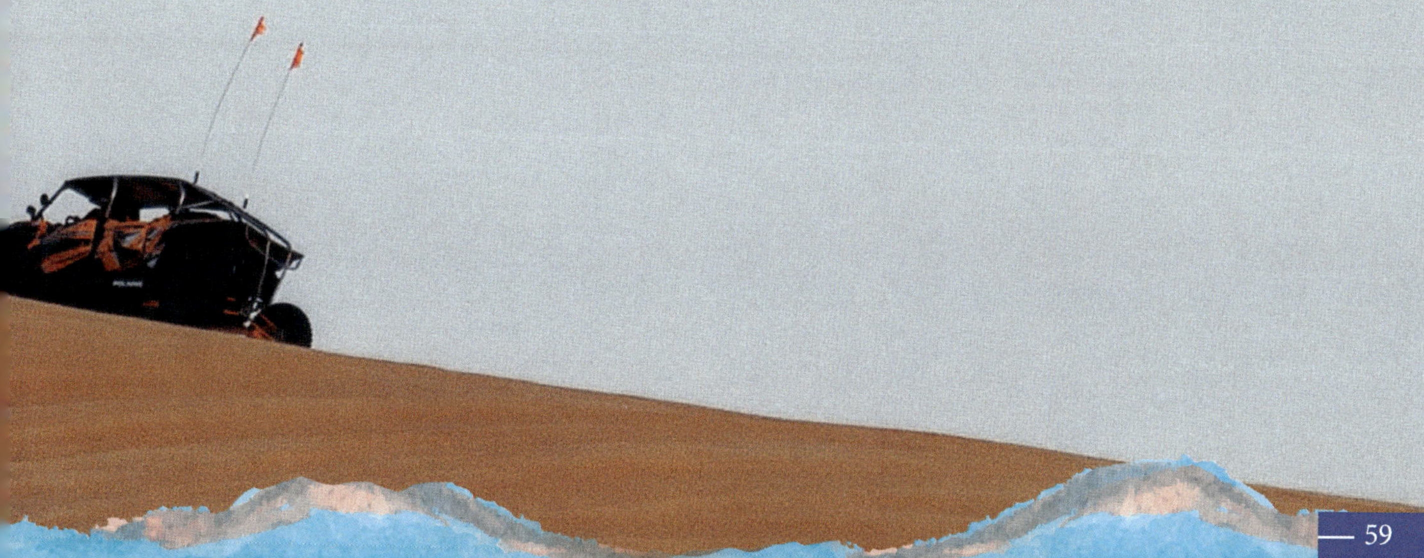

Predatory Spirits in the Womb

What if the enemy can capture the emotions of your soul while you are still in your mother's womb? What if he launches a scheme against you that cannot be discovered by searching your memory banks? These embedded memories lie in the quiet archives of your soul and make regular impromptu appearances at crucial moments in your life. Sometimes they will overwhelm you with fear and anxiety.

At other times memories can leave you emotionally undone and vulnerable. Alternatively, these memories could run as an emotional background program to all your life experiences. The result will be a lingering fear or the sense that there is always a dark cloud around the next corner. In summary, these schemes cannot be detected by memory, but they affect every aspect of your existence.

If you have suffered womb trauma, you may find yourself behaving in ways that have no reasonable explanation - always covering your vulnerability by any means possible and trying to run ahead of every imagined storm. The wounds created in the womb have several themes, including rejection, fear and abandonment.

These are not only powerful emotional reactions, but they are spirits that can follow you all the days of your life. This would leave you permanently trapped and often paralysed to take action. Most wounds created in the soul of the unborn child are due to conversations between parents and significant others. Parents are the spiritual custodians of the unborn child. **When a child's soul is left unprotected by the immaturity of parents, the enemy has easy access to the child** - traumatising the baby in the womb and setting up a vulnerability pattern that's virtually undetectable in adulthood.

Generational Spirits

Other spirits that operate in the womb are generational spirits. These spirits relate to things that happened before you were born. They are linked to interactions people had around you, while you were still in the womb. The enemy is aware of everything that happened to you in the womb and uses this information to trigger you at various points in your life.

If you dealt with rejection in the womb, the enemy will use any opportunity in the present time to bring back this emotion in your current relationships.

He knows how to trigger you and get you to feel waves of rejection from the smallest acts and words. In general, your reactions will be out of proportion to the circumstances you encounter. Once emotions are triggered, old files are opened. Decisions are made on raw emotion and not under the guidance of the Holy Spirit.

This often leads to conflict, strife and a breakdown of important relationships.

The enemy is now in charge and releases his power over your decision. However, if we ask, God always comes to our aid with the gifts of discernment, deliverance, healing and restoration.

"Your Memory May Forget, But Your Emotions Remember"

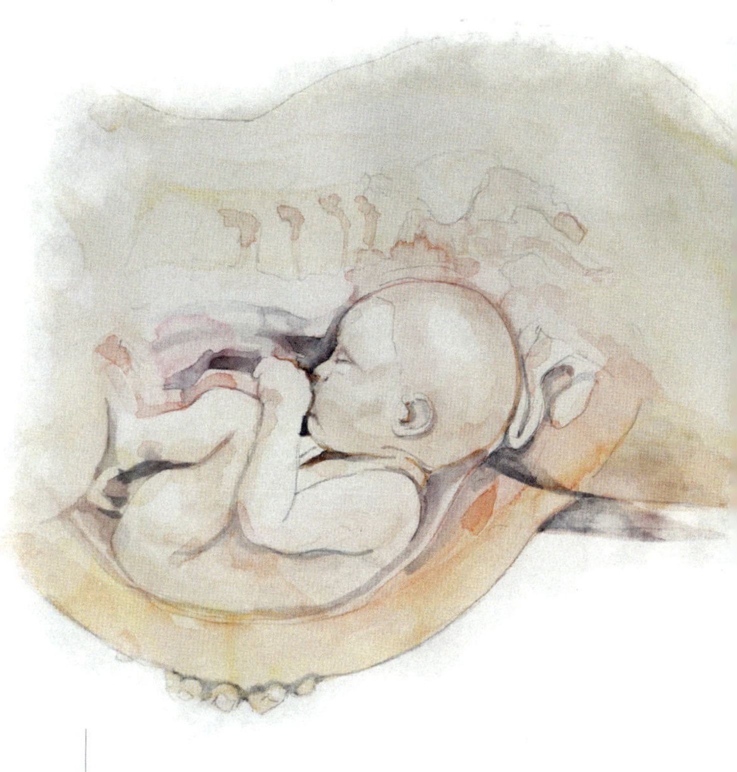

The Womb to Womb Encounter: Jesus Christ and John the Baptist

Jesus and John 'met' for the first time while they were still in the wombs of their mothers. A recently pregnant Mary went to visit her cousin Elizabeth who was six months pregnant with John. In the gospel of Luke, Chapter 1, verse 41 it is written that: 'When Elizabeth heard Mary's greeting... the baby leapt in the womb'. It was a leaping of joy in the soul of baby John, for he was in the presence of the Lord.

Thirty years later, John was baptising hundreds of people in the River Jordan. There is no biblical record of any contact between Jesus and John for thirty years. The scriptures tell us that Jesus comes to John to be baptised, but John initially refuses and says: 'I need to be baptised by you'. However John relents, and baptises Jesus. Jesus is then taken immediately by the Holy Spirit into the wilderness for forty days to be tempted by the devil. On day forty-one or so, when Jesus passes John again, he says *'Behold the lamb of God who takes away the sin of the world'. (John, Chapter 1, Verse 29).*

The critical question in this biblical narrative is why did John initially refuse to baptise Jesus? John himself said: *'I would not have known him' (John Chapter 1, Verses 31-33).* The answer is that after thirty years, 'the baby leapt in the womb a second time'. John had experienced the same emotion of joy he had in the womb of his mother - for the second time.

This tells us that the womb is a place of interaction, memory and emotion in the child. The story of Jesus and John in the womb shows that womb experiences can predispose people to certain behaviours thirty years later. Many of us will not know or understand the origins of these experiences in our own lives, but will live with the positive or negative effects of them.

Personal Reflection

Your Womb History

Your time in the womb of your mother is the seed and cradle of the tree of your life. Writing about this time most often entails seeking information from your parents, family members and their close friends. Take time to have meaningful conversations about your early history and record the information below:

- What was the first response of your father to the news that your mother was pregnant with you?

- What was the emotional state of your mother during her pregnancy? Was she anxious, fearful, unsupported, depressed or isolated, or was it a time of peace and celebration?

- Were you a planned or unplanned pregnancy or the consequence of an affair, premarital sex or sexual abuse of your mother?

- What were the financial circumstances of both your parents when you were in the womb of your mother? Did they have sufficient finances or did you represent another mouth to feed?

- Was there ever talk of aborting you or giving you up for adoption? What were the circumstances and outcome of these conversations?

- What was the spiritual condition of both your parents? Were they grounded in the same faith or did they have diverse belief systems? Was there religious conflict between the extended families?

- What were the societal and global conditions during the time of your mother's pregnancy? Example: war, migration, genocide or a global pandemic.

Personal Reflection

Personal Reflection

PART 1

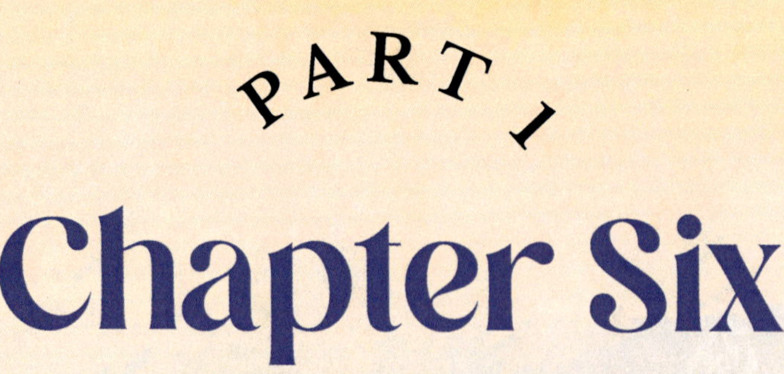

Chapter Six

Ratification And Vows

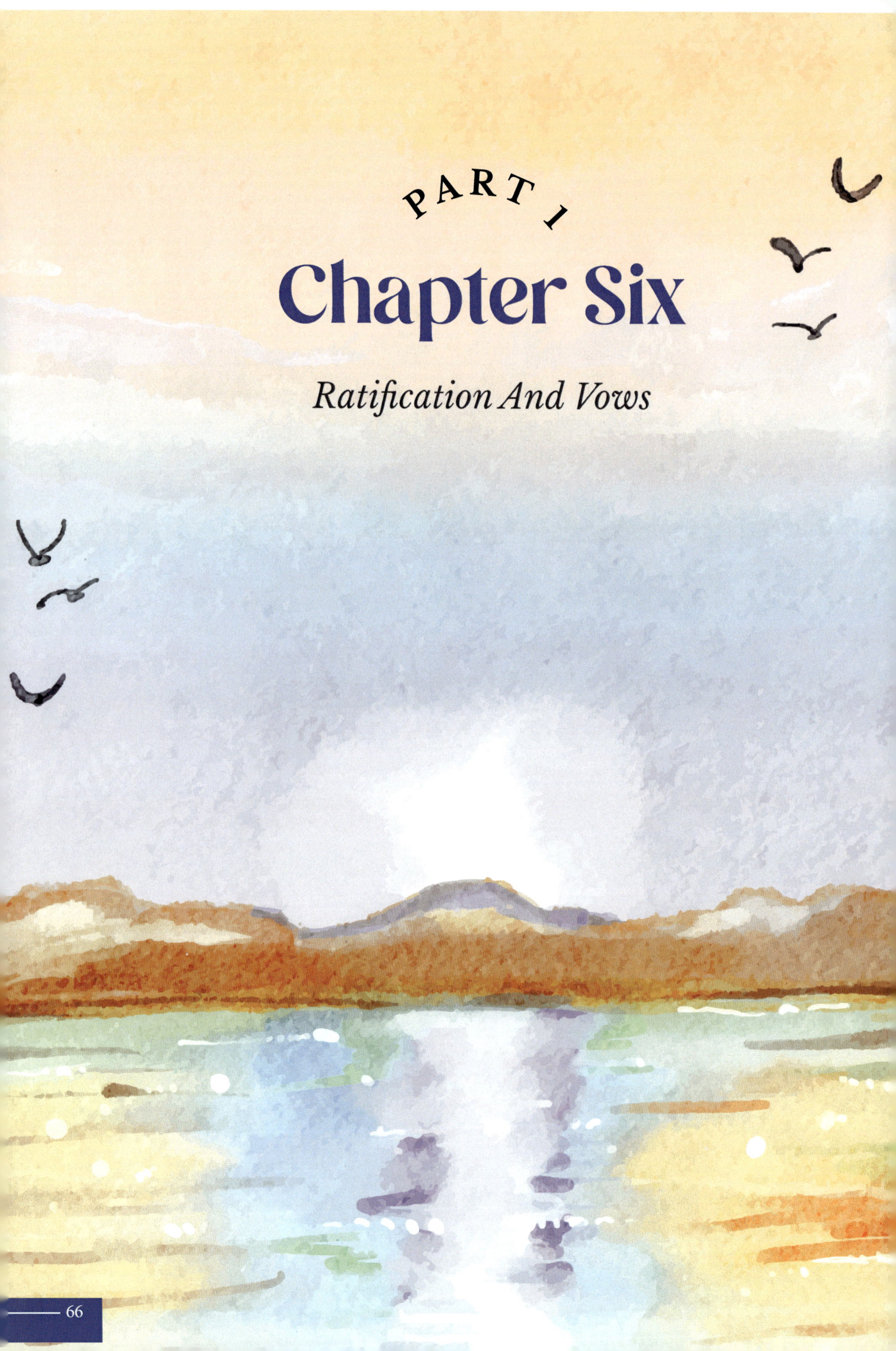

Raya's Ridicule

As far back as Raya could remember she felt unwanted. In therapy she discovered that her discarding and rejection began in the womb of her mother. Her parents were unwed at the time of Raya's conception. Her grandparents were conservative and emotionally neglected both mother and child.

She grew up in a strict home with her single mother, grandparents and three uncles. The family took every opportunity to remind her that she was a burden and millstone around their necks. Her father was prevented from visiting and communicating with her.

Raya had a desperate need to belong somewhere or with someone. At eighteen she met her father for the first time and he showered her with gifts and affection. His new wife saw Raya as a threat and thwarted further visits. Her father died suddenly a year later and Raya's sense of aloneness and abandonment expanded.

At nineteen she married a teacher and longed to have a place to call home. She soon learnt that he was an abusive alcoholic. He took self-satisfaction in taunting her with the words: *'Nobody wants you'.*

Over time Raya began to believe and agree with the lies spoken to her and they became her default setting. She began a slow journey of healing and focused on reclaiming her true identity as a child of the living God.

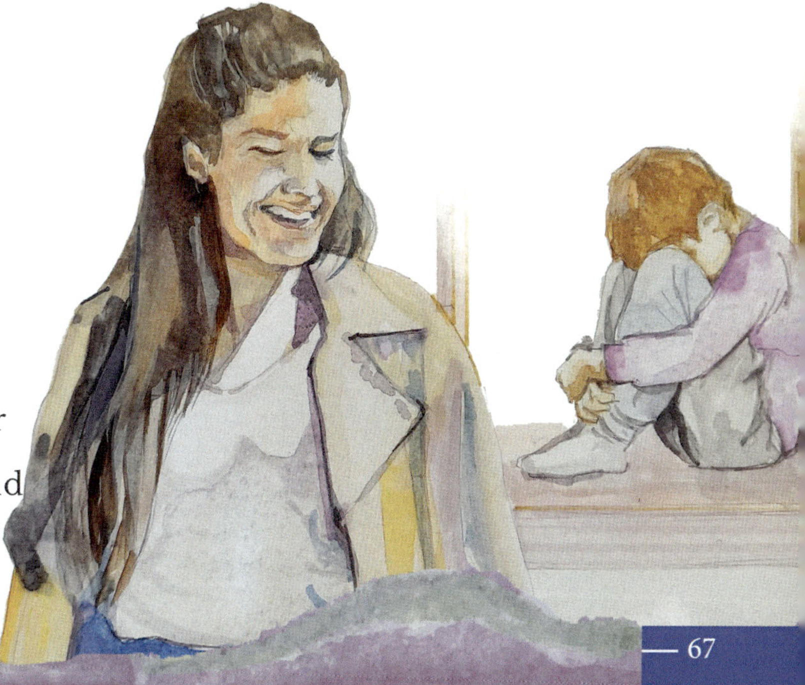

Chapter Six

Ratification

To *'ratify'* means to approve, sanction or confirm a matter. The notion of ratification is crucial in distinguishing between the actions of others towards us and our own actions towards ourselves. Raya began to engage a process of forgiveness in therapy. Forgiveness is an essential core of all healing journeys.

She forgave her parents, family members and finally herself. This was an arduous undertaking. In her healing work, she discovered that she had believed the lies her caregivers spoke over her and agreed with their false conclusions about her personhood and identity. Raya had ratified the lies spoken about her.

When a person ratifies a behaviour, independent of the actions of others, they provide a legal basis by which demonic spirits can oppress them. Ratification often happens spontaneously and automatically. You are now aware that the enemy can install lies in the emotions of an unborn child. These lies can be successively confirmed by others from that time onwards into the teenage years.

The circumstances of life are now

Ratification Continued...

viewed through false lenses and become a vicious entrapment. As the person approaches adulthood, they will either do or say something that moves them from the actions of others, to what they accept as being true about themselves.

In summary, during the process of ratification, a person receives the lie as if were the truth. As time progresses, the person begins to act in a way that mutates that lie into a personal truth. Typically, the person does not reflect on the past or examines situations and the behaviour of self and others.

They simply continue accepting the lie as the truth. At this point in time they have handed their enemy - unwittingly and unknowingly - the right to oppress them, because they have agreed with the lie. Raya came to agree with the lie that she was a burden and that no one wanted her.

Vows

Have you ever made statements that began with the words *'I swear'* or *'I will never'*?

If you did, you have made a vow to others or yourself. A vow is a solemn promise to complete a particular task. A vow is also binding and specific. Inaccurate vows turn us into slaves. Raya vowed to never talk to certain family members again. She also vowed never to trust her mother.

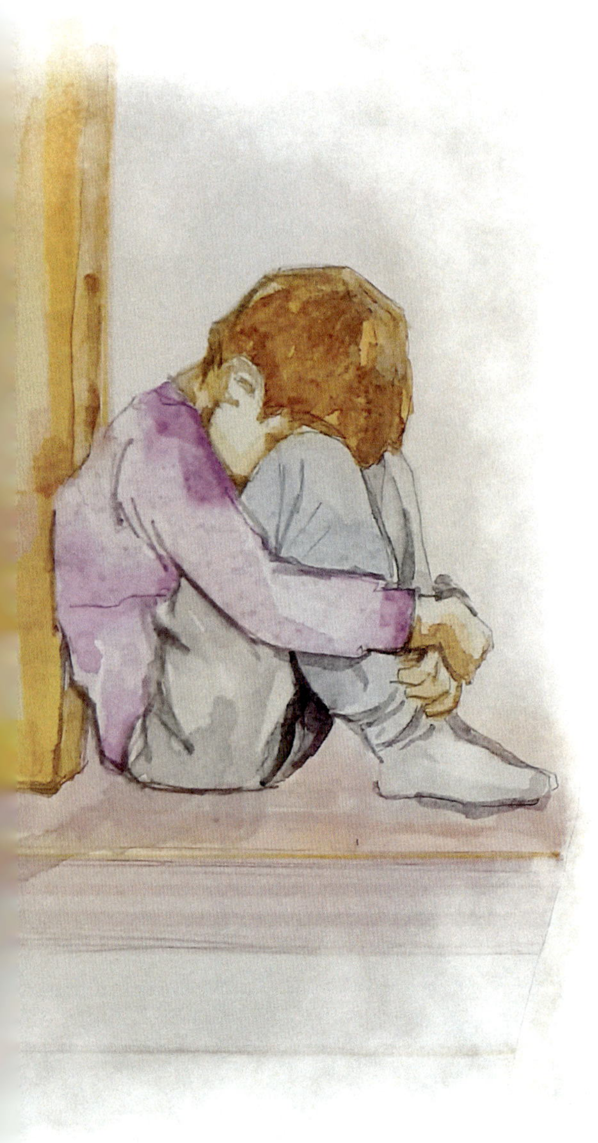

It was her way of putting distance between herself and those she viewed as having caused her harm. However, she was faced with a dilemma when her only son insisted on inviting her biological family to his wedding. Raya understood the importance of his request and did not want her personal feelings to place a strain on his wedding day. She now had to renege on the promise she had made never to see them again.

In addition to this, Raya also vowed to never go through a divorce or challenge her husband's bullying. She had made a vow to never stand up to his abuse and to avoid all conflict. This meant she had to endure daily emotional abuse and alcoholic rages. Vows become statements that the enemy uses over time to torment the vow-maker. Raya felt guilty and enslaved by her own vows and she began to spiral into anxiety and despair. The enemy had her trapped.

The Bondage of Vows

Vows also take the form of one person putting another into bondage. This happens by getting the other person to take on responsibility for which they have no authority, ability, maturity or resources. If the person accepts these conditions, they will eventually feel like a failure. My patient Ajax is twenty years old and comes from a family where his two older brothers are addicted to cocaine.

This meant that Ajax was constantly on edge wondering when they would disappear for the weekend. It became Ajax's responsibility to fetch his siblings from crack houses in violent neighbourhoods. I encouraged Ajax to tell me about the intrinsic vows he had unwittingly made about his siblings. He adapted the Bible: *'I am my brothers' keeper'.* Once this rolled off his tongue, a light bulb went off in his brain. He realised his inability to say no to his parents, who expected him to be on standby for his siblings. The enemy had trapped Ajax for years and made him live in a state of constant anxiety. **The recognition of his erroneous vow-making accelerated his healing journey.**

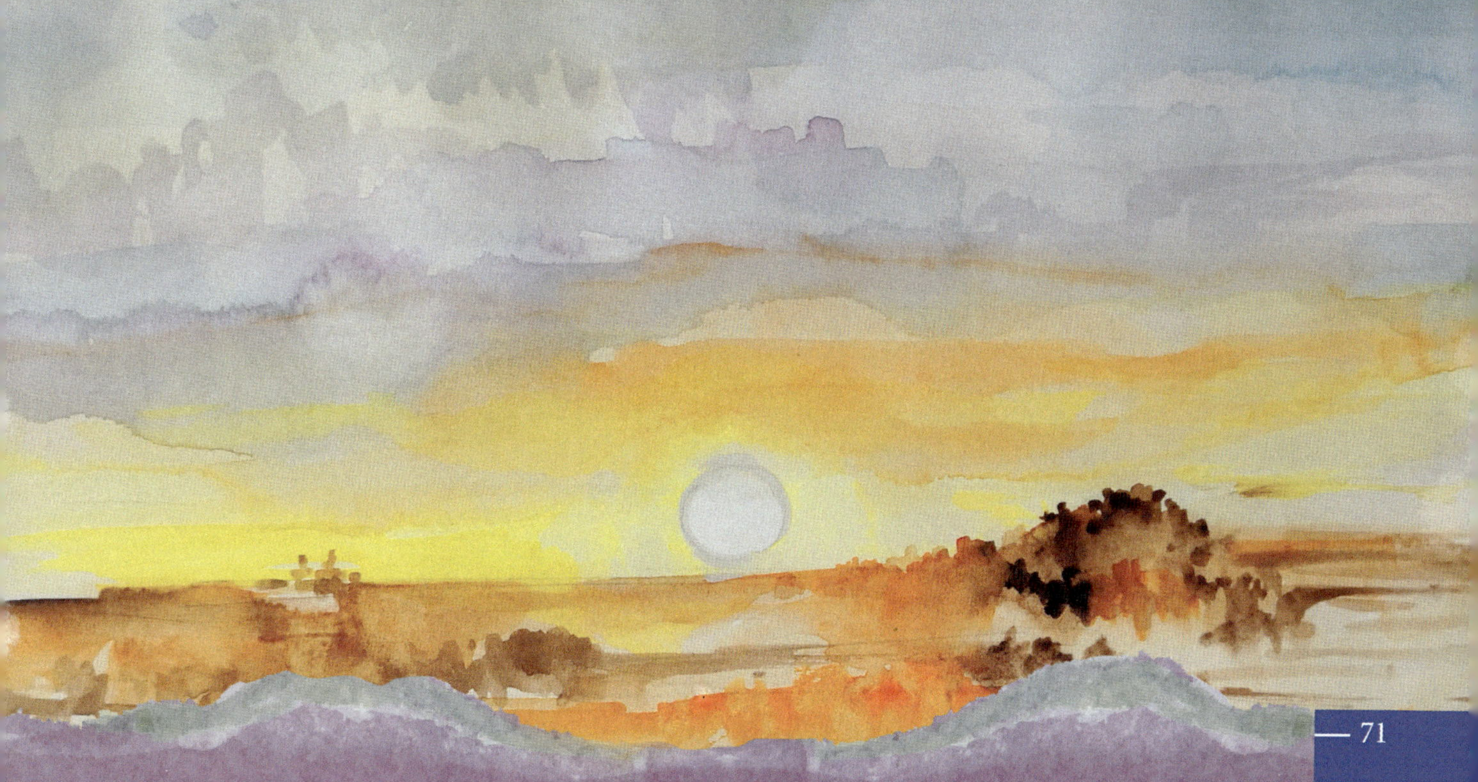

Personal Reflection

Ratification

We have learnt that the process of ratification involves believing the lies we have heard about who we are. Reflect and record some of the lies you believed about yourself and ratified since childhood.

Vows

Many of us make vows without the full knowledge and awareness of what is required to fulfill them. Make a list of your vows that began with 'I swear' or '*I will never...*'.

1. ____

____

2. ____

____

3. ____

____

Personal Reflection

Personal Reflection

Removing The Blockages

A Practical Cure

In this final part of the Workbook, a remedy in the form of practical cure is provided to cast out any and all demonic spirits from your soul. Find a quiet place to engage this critical part of your healing journey. There is nothing to fear as a child of God, as it is your right and spiritual inheritance to be freed and made whole. **Be courageous in claiming and living out your healing.**

You are going to be guided through the following sections:

1. Sonship and Spiritual Authority

2. Freedom through Forgiveness

3. Blockage Removal Administration

(by Dr. Sam Soleyn)

Let's Begin...

Chapter Seven

Sonship And Spiritual Authority

Chapter Seven

Understanding Sonship

God created humanity and the world to put on display the nature of His love. When Adam separated himself from his Father, he changed from a son to a spiritual orphan. Sonship is the most significant concept that God wants every human being to grasp, understand, and walk in. God is love, (1 John 4:8, 4:16), and He created sons (male and female) to show His love and glory - both to them and through them. We know that God was creating sons because He made humankind in 'our own image, according to our likeness (not a physical, but a spiritual personality and a moral likeness), and He let them rule over the fish of the sea and the birds of the air, over the cattle, and over all of the earth...' (Genesis 1:26).

Just as progeny resembles the father in the natural, God made sons to represent Him in the spiritual sense. Salvation is part of God's plan, but it is not the ultimate purpose. The supreme purpose is to have sons who truly represent the Father. These sons will rule righteously, according to the Father's eternal standards, and will truly understand that they are spirit beings contained in flesh.

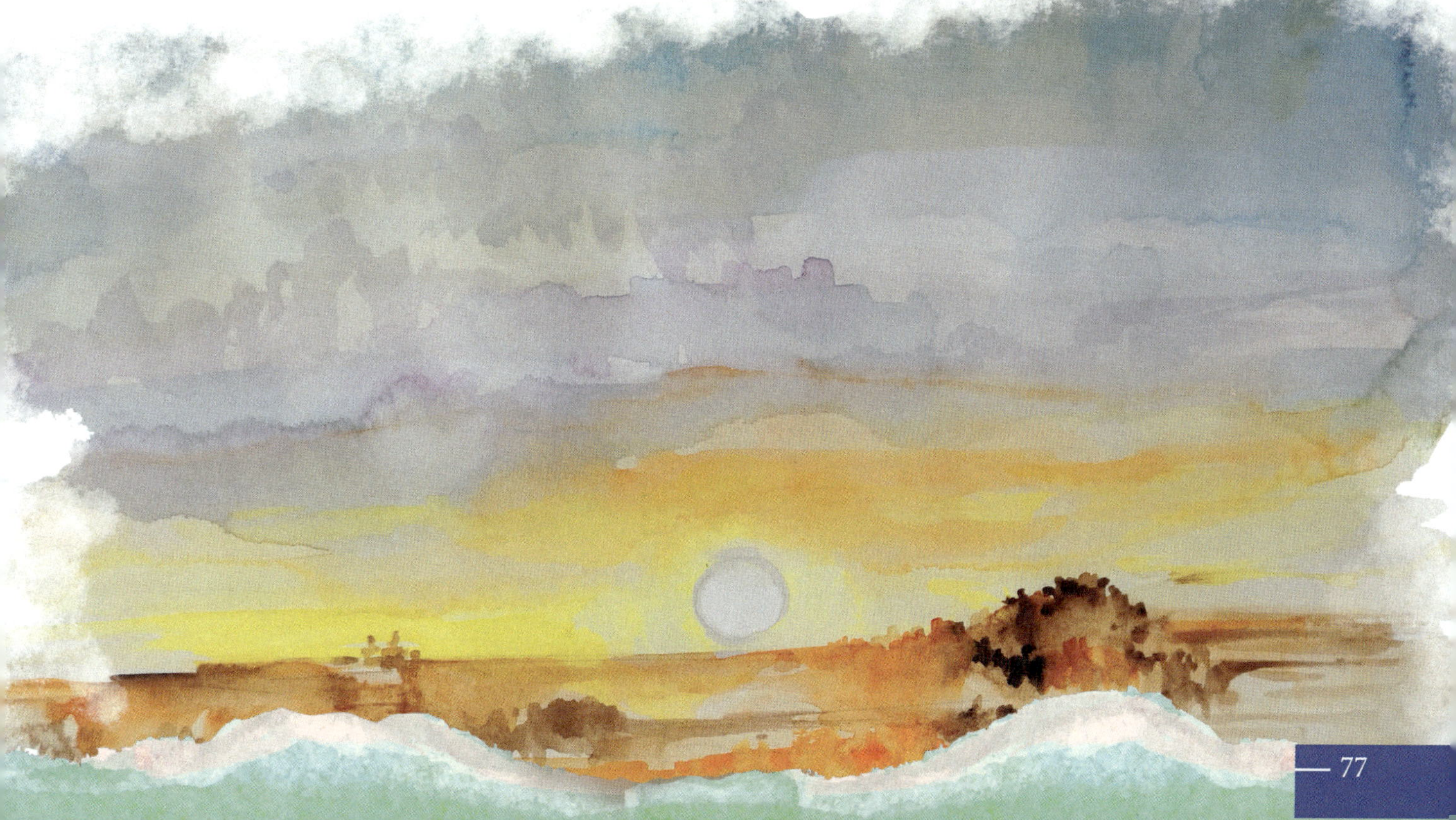

Spirit to spirit

When you speak of a son of God, you are speaking about someone whose Father is a Spirit. Hence, the son of God is a spirit being contained in the flesh. When God breathed life into man (Genesis 2:17); He imparted into man a spirit of His own - so that man could communicate with God, Spirit to spirit. This singular aspect is what separates man from all creation, including the angelic.

> *When we grow in our desire to really know Christ, our spirits become progressively more active in fellowship with the Holy Spirit.*

We come to love Him more, to obey Him, and to put His will ahead of our own. That is the point where we begin to become considered a mature son of God. But we do not become that immediately, once we receive Christ. There is a process that we walk through before being considered mature. John 1:12 says 'as many as receive Him, to them He gave the right to become sons of God'. There is a transformation that occurs in the maturing process, that results in us becoming mature sons of God.

Stages of Sonship

God gives us the natural to understand the spiritual. In the natural, we start out as a child and go through a maturation process to become adults. The same is true for the sons of God. The different levels of development can be seen throughout the bible. In the New Testament, the original Greek translation gives us a clearer understanding of the word 'son'. Son can cover the spectrum of meaning from a newborn infant (nepios), to a little child (paidion), or a teenager (teknon), or a young adult (neaniskos) and finally a fully mature son (huios) - who accurately represents the Father.

A Spiritual Father

This maturing process is best accomplished with the help of a spiritual father.

A spiritual father is a mature man of God, who is able to mentor and guide you in your spiritual growth. A good example of this relationship is seen between Paul and Timothy. Timothy was not Paul's natural son.

Acts 16:1 states that Timothy was the son of a Jewish woman and a Greek father, yet Paul referred to Timothy as 'my child in the Lord', (1 Corinthians 4:17) and my child in the faith, (1 Timothy 1:1 and 1 Timothy 1:18).

The spiritual father teaches a son, to see how he or she is ruled by their soul and their worldly ways. He helps them transition from the rule of their soul in their lives, to the rule of the Spirit of God. This teaches them to go from relying on their reason, their emotions, and their worldly ways for provision and protection to relying on God Himself - as they learn to trust what the Spirit is showing them.

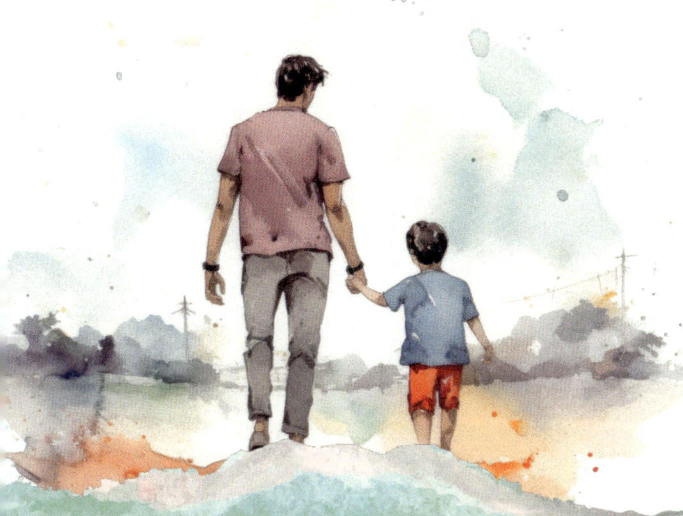

The spiritual father comes alongside the son to teach and assist. He settles the emotions of the soul of the son because the soul is not a reliable instrument for faith towards God. He explains the role of suffering that is necessary for maturing.

This process is designed to limit and restrict, the input of the soul in determining the true nature of reality. This allows our spirit to be the dominant lead in our lives.

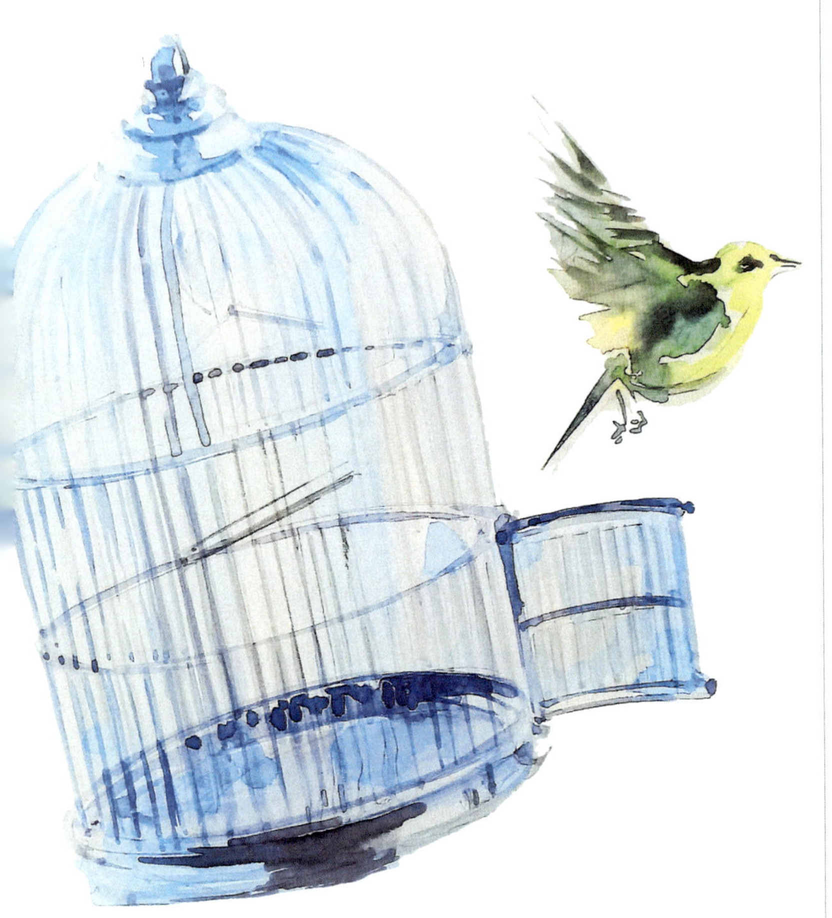

Ephesians 4:8 states that Christ Jesus gave certain gifts to men. These gifts are listed as apostles, prophets, evangelists, pastors and teachers. Jeremiah 3:15 states: 'Then I will give you shepherds after My own heart, who will feed you with knowledge and understanding'.

A spiritual father is a shepherd, who gives care and oversight to those who have committed themselves and chosen to follow God's precepts.

Chapter Seven

The most important aspect of a true spiritual father is that he rules for the benefit of the son. He also teaches sons to rule righteously - in the same way that Jesus did. Jesus lived on the earth in a manner distinct from all other humans.

He showed us that it is possible to hear God and to walk in divine communion moment by moment. Jesus' life is a blueprint of the life God intended for us - his sons. He has made available, to all humanity, the opportunity to be reconciled to God the Father. Jesus also showed us how to dismantle and overthrow every demonic deception and scheme.

He reintroduced the authority of heaven into the earth. *This authority is known as the Kingdom of God and supports each of us as we overcome the schemes of the enemy and live out our divine purpose.*

Today understand that demonic spirits only have a place of authority in your life because:
- *You gave a demonic spirit a door to enter your soul OR*
- *Someone who had authority to act on your behalf did not do so effectively and left you exposed to demonic entrapment.*

So remember....

You are in Christ and your enemy has no legitimate authority over you. The youngest son in the family of God, who has the awareness of these aspects of the Kingdom of God, can speak to the demonic spirit and it has to obey. This spiritual truth must become embedded in your being as you evict every spirit hidden in the emotions of your soul.

Know that when we appeal to God to free us, 'Deliver us from the evil one,' is part of what we call the Lord's Prayer (Matthew, chapter 6, verse 13). He will respond. God will not allow the enemy to have any legitimate authority over you. Stolen authority will never meet with the approval of our righteous God.

Personal Reflection

Your Journey of Sonship

This chapter identified five stages of sonship : a newborn infant (nepios), a little child (paidion), a teenager (teknon), a young adult (neaniskos) and a fully mature son (huios). **Write a few notes on your journey of sonship - your current level of development and the previous stages you have been through.**

Personal Reflection

Personal Reflection

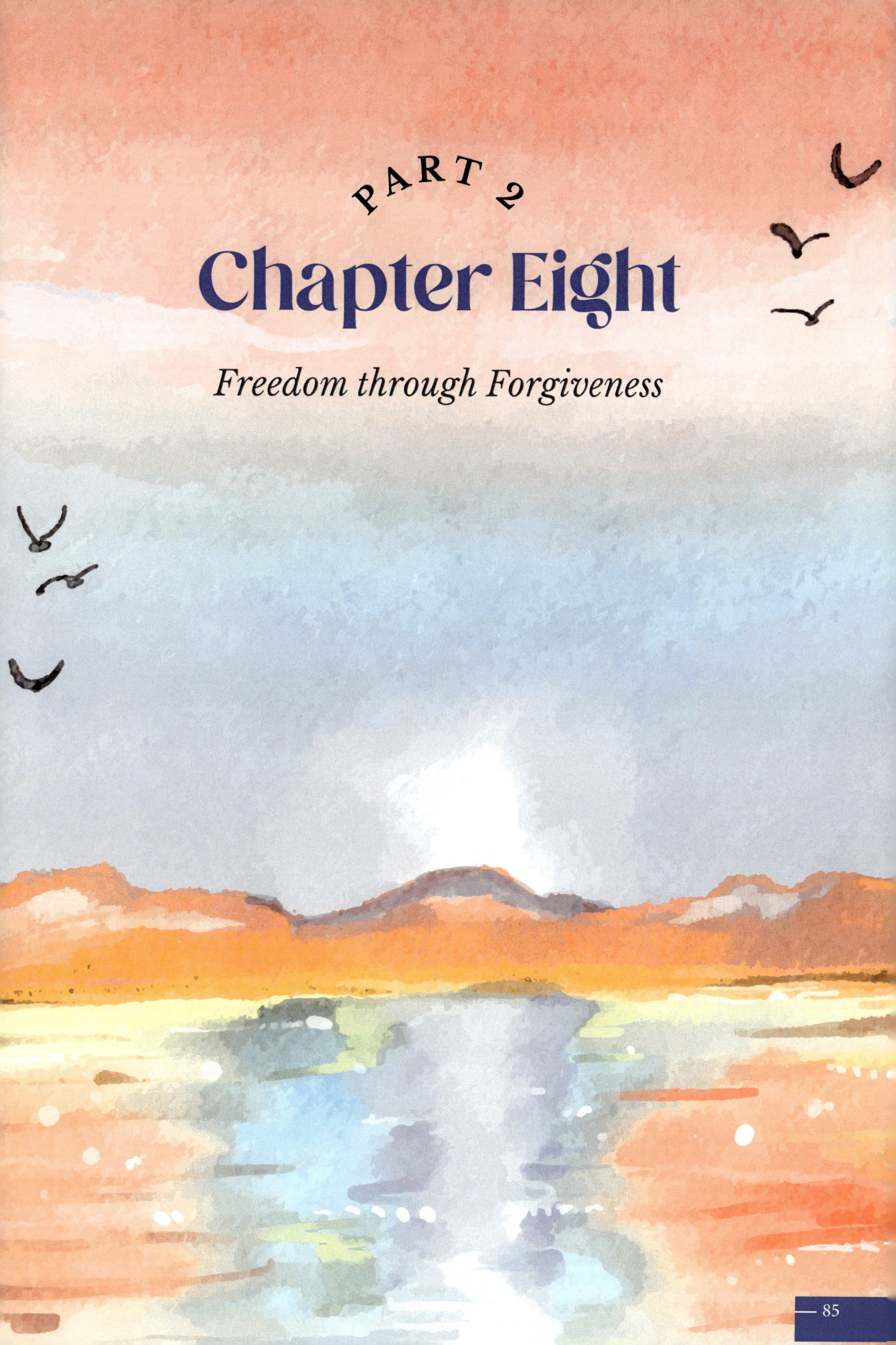

PART 2
Chapter Eight
Freedom through Forgiveness

Invisible Handcuffs

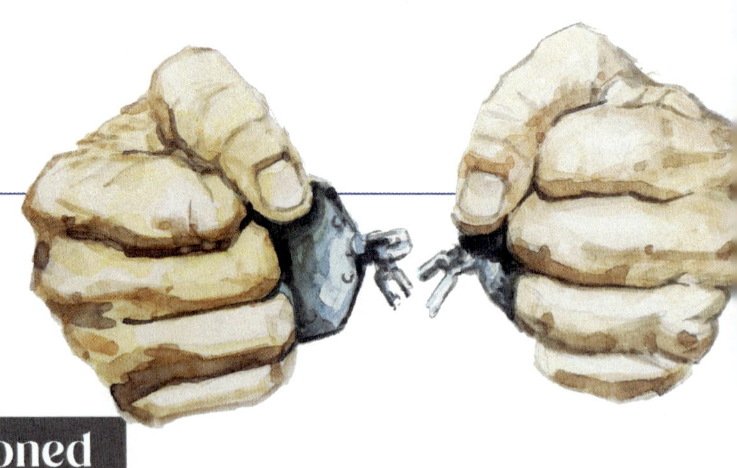

Imagine a pair of metal handcuffs.

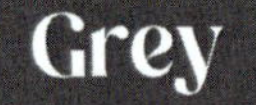

Grey　**Cold**　**Imprisoned**

Now imagine one cuff on your right wrist and the other cuff on the left wrist of the person you need to forgive. Everywhere you go, the person goes with you - shackled together. Unforgiveness keeps you hostage to those that have hurt and harmed you. Forgiveness is the key that unlocks the handcuffs and sets you free from the chains of your past. **When you choose to forgive, your enemy has no legal ground to keep you captive.**

There are three categories of forgiveness for your healing:

The **first category** is to forgive ancestors up to and including your parents. These are your caregivers who had authority over you but failed to exercise their rule correctly. Their lack of spiritual covering and protection allowed the enemy to come in and torment you. Forgiving them cancels the claim of the enemy's authority - because there is now an acknowledgement of their breach of duty towards you. This breach is a sin against you.

The **second category** of forgiveness is towards people whose actions, activities, and behaviour were sinful towards you. This is a catch-all category, and the Spirit of discernment will help you identify exactly what was done and by whom. As you reflect, you will also come to understand the impact of their attitudes and stance against you.

The **third category** of forgiveness is receiving forgiveness from God by repenting to God for vows and ratifications made by yourself. This is when you agreed with the lies of your enemy. In believing the lies, you committed two sins. The first sin was against God because you accepted the lie that God made you in a condition of brokenness - incapable of carrying His presence.
It is vitally important to acknowledge that it is a sin against God when you believe lies against yourself. This is because this sin separates and distances you from God.

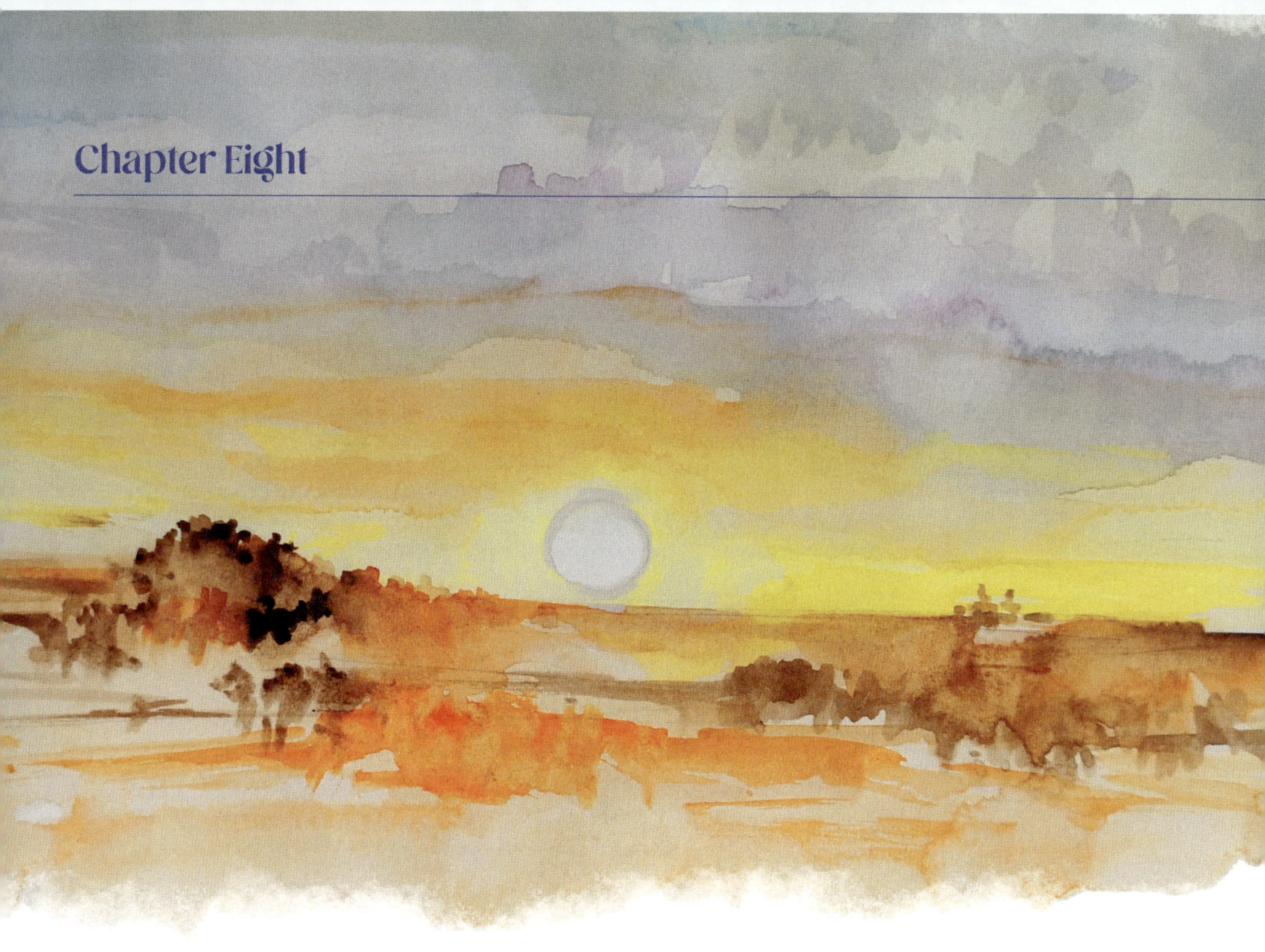

Believing the Lie

The second sin you committed was against yourself because you inserted a lie in the place of truth. From God's point of view you believed something false about yourself. Your entrapment is that you continued to see yourself as damaged and beyond the reach of God. When this happens in your life, you see God as unwilling to rise in your circumstances and shower you with an increased measure of faith, hope and love.

When you confess your sins against God and against yourself, you are guaranteed forgiveness. Once forgiven, your enemy has no authority to prosecute, judge, condemn, or occupy space in your emotions. He has become a trespasser. Now, he is no longer a fierce, predatory enemy. Instead, he is sitting in the seat of the condemned, awaiting sentencing.

Personal Reflection

Forgiveness

When you forgive you set yourself free. Forgiveness is not condoning, absolving or downplaying the sins perpetrated against you. Instead, it is purposefully acknowledging the wrongs and intentionally choosing to pardon the people who have harmed you.

Make a list of the people you need to forgive.

1.

2.

3.

Personal Reflection

Personal Reflection

Chapter Nine

Blockage Removal Administration
By Dr. Sam Soleyn

Casting out spirits

In this portion of the Workbook, you have the opportunity to undertake a practical process of casting out all demonic spirits embedded in the emotions of your soul.

This is known as blockage removal administration of grace. It formed the major theme of a conference held in Cape Town, South Africa. The purpose of this process is to free your soul from all demonic influences. This will then ensure that your soul is once again able to come under the rule of your spirit, which is under the authority of the Holy Spirit.

When this transpires, the mind of your spirit will govern the mind of your soul and the thoughts of God will become your thoughts. Further, the Kingdom of God will now come into your time and space and fill you with righteousness, peace and joy in the Holy Spirit.

This will result in you rising up and maturing in your sonship and becoming the 'Zion of God'. *You will be the place out of which God shines in the earth and you will fulfill your destiny.*

Chapter Nine

Let's Begin

We are going to cast out two of the most common spirits. Number one is the spirit of rejection, or abandonment as often is the manifestation of it. The other is the spirit of fear. Now, this is a beginning. It is not an end. It is a beginning. Take note of how this is done, and whenever the enemy arises within your perimeter, apply the Truth, in either this fashion, or a fashion similar to it. You may well need the help of a spiritual father who watches over your soul in order to take up what was lost to you after the demonic has been expelled.

The word for spirit is the word, "pneuma" or wind. When a spirit leaves, it is not uncommon to experience an expulsion of air, or the ringing of your ears, or physical tensioning and release. If any of that occurs to you, that is just the spirit leaving.

Nothing may actually happen, but because you are exercising divine authority, you are removing the authority of your enemy to control you. You are taking back the possession of your soul in order to give it willingly and intentionally to the rule of the spirit.

Let's begin by dealing with one of the most common ways that these spirits come in, which is the neglect of parents or the ignorance of parents. We will begin by forgiving your parents. *As you do this, it might come to you with clarity which of your parents you need to forgive.*

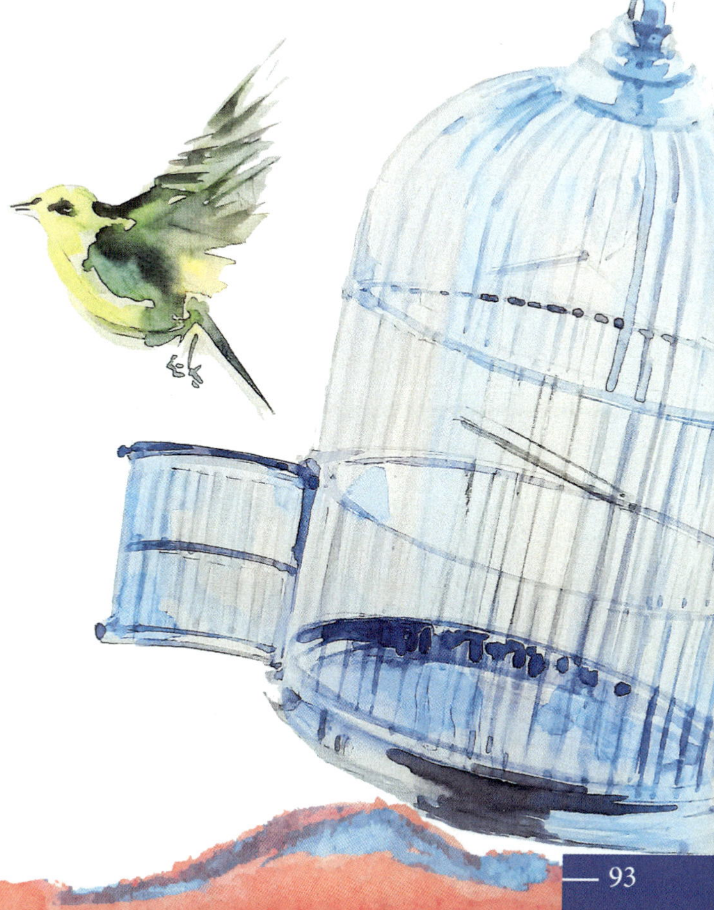

Chapter Nine

It may not be both, but it may be. They may have been in collusion in some fashion, unintentionally, most likely. The failure of their authority was a sin against you. As you forgive them, we are going to specify that you are forgiving them of their sins against you, which has caused great harm to you, harm in the form of distress.

Then, the next thing we will do is I will lead you through a declaration of repentance for agreeing with the lie. That cuts off an independent cause that the enemy may assert against you. When you have done both things, forgiven those who have trespassed or repented of your own endorsement, then the legal ground of your enemy has been retaken. So, we will specifically demand our rights as the sons of God against our enemy, and we will demand that our enemy leaves us. And he will leave you. This is not hope or wish; this is the exercise of the authority of God in which we have been fully enfranchised. I will lead you through the first section, which is forgiveness.

We will start with a statement; just repeat after me.

- I make the following declarations from my position as a son of God
- I choose to forgive my parents for their sins against me. They failed to guard me in my infancy from the ravages of my enemy.
- As a result, I have suffered for most of my life with the consequences of their failures.
- I specifically forgive them for words and actions that produced an opening in my soul to the spirit of rejection and the spirit of abandonment.
- I further forgive them for enabling the spirit of fear to invade my soul's emotions.
- These failures have been hurtful and harmful, and have robbed me of life.
- It is with the full knowledge of this that I choose to forgive my parents for their sins against me.
- Furthermore, I recognise that I have believed the lie, and by that I have empowered my enemy against me. I acknowledge that that is a sin against myself.

Chapter Nine

- I ask God to forgive me of this sin and to cleanse me from the authority that I gave to my enemy.

- This is my declaration and my confession of sin, made this day before the throne of God, before men, and before angels. In the Name of Jesus, I so declare. *Amen.*

- Your enemy, now, has no authority against you.

> *Now comes the fun part: Taking back what is yours.*
> *I want you to say, raise your hands:*

- I reject and I renounce the spirit of rejection and its companion, the spirit of abandonment.

- I now command them to leave my body, to exit my soul.

- I reject and I renounce the spirit of fear. I now command it to depart from my soul, in the Name and by the authority of the Lord Jesus Christ. *Amen.*

- Now, I am going to make a declaration on your behalf. Just relax.

- To the spirit of abandonment, to the spirit of rejection, and to the spirit of fear, I declare on behalf of the Lord and on behalf of His people here tonight, you have no authority in their lives. No more! Now be gone, in the

- Name of Jesus. Be gone! The Lord rebukes you. Be gone! In the Name of Jesus. *Amen*

When he tries to come back, it will not come back inside of your perimeter. He will try to reason with you from outside. Between the time they make an appeal to you and the time you have to answer the appeal, the Holy Spirit will show you what to say. When you declare it, you will continue to perfect the victory that you have been given tonight.

I commend you to God and to the Word of His grace that is able to build you up and to establish you among the sanctified. *Amen.*

The Way Forward

It's the relationship that heals

When I was discovering my path as a twenty-something novice psychotherapist, I came across a quote by Irvin Yalom, a renowned psychiatrist, that read: 'It's the relationship that heals, the relationship that heals, the relationship that heals — my professional rosary.' This perceptive observation became the foundational stone of my healing work with patients. As clinical psychologists we are astute in assessing symptoms and formulating diagnosis; however, I have found that the quality and depth of the therapeutic relationship is the heartbeat of the healing journey.

For many patients, it is the first authentic human bond that is safe, honest and free from rejection and abandonment.

The relationship between you and your Heavenly Father is the true location of deep profound healing. It is this relationship bathed in His presence, divine power and eternal love that transforms you back into who He created you to be. Today, understand that regardless of your inconsistencies, shifting attitudes, and general changes in human nature, nothing can change the love of the Father towards you.

This love is divine and eternally the same towards you. It is this supernatural relationship between you and the Father that heals all wounds and brings restoration to your life. Let it become your daily quest to explore the scriptures and dwell in the presence of the Lord.

Watching over your Soul

A final recommendation is that you subject yourself to the delegated authority that God has placed in your life, who is capable of watching over your soul. This will be a spiritual father or elder in the faith. This earthly authority is your early-warning system and spiritual covering. It also helps you, not only to formulate how you may destroy your enemy's attack against you, but it serves to remind you of what God has already done and what you now are positioned to do as it regards your enemy.

In essence, while you are learning to become familiar with new emotions (that had been denied to you for so long), submit yourself to the person that God has placed in authority over you and trust their words.

Your awareness of the schemes of your enemy and your ability to function to resist the enemy are still new; whereas the person watching over your soul knows you and the strategies of your enemy.

A spiritual father can guide you through this process, at a time when you are learning how to engage all that you have been given back.

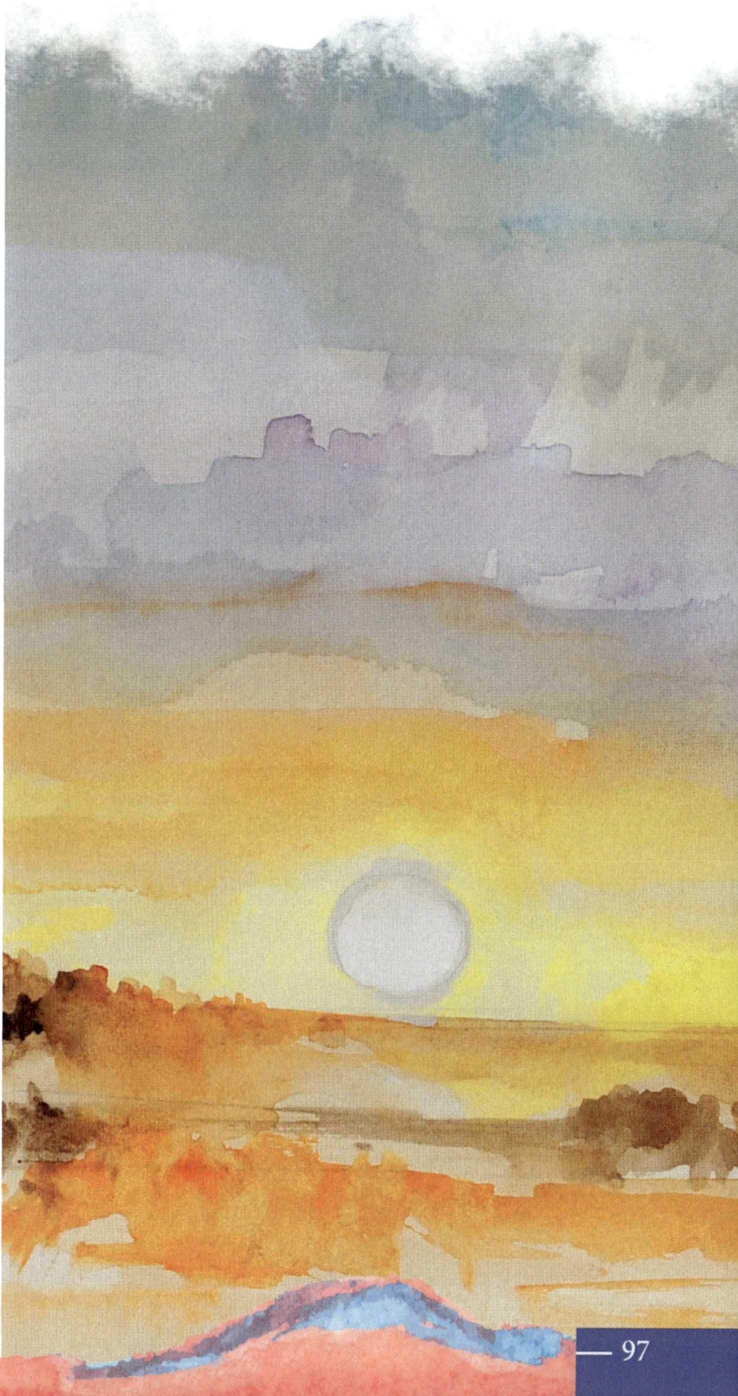

Know your Authority

Lastly, may the Lord bless you with the Spirit of understanding, that you might know your authority in Christ over your enemy. Further, may God free you from all the harm that the works of the devil have inflicted upon your soul. May the Lord rescue you entirely from every scheme of your enemy, as He continues the process of saving your soul. This entire healing of trauma journey is about saving your soul. It is the process of the salvation of the soul - the rescue of your soul from the control of your enemy. Thereafter, it is the step of the re-positioning of your soul under the rule of your spirit. This is taking place so that when your spirit hears God, your soul might agree - and together with your spirit ruling your soul, your soul might execute the works of God as you are led to within your body. *This will result in your spirit, soul, and body being sanctified and set apart for the purposes of God thoroughly and completely.*

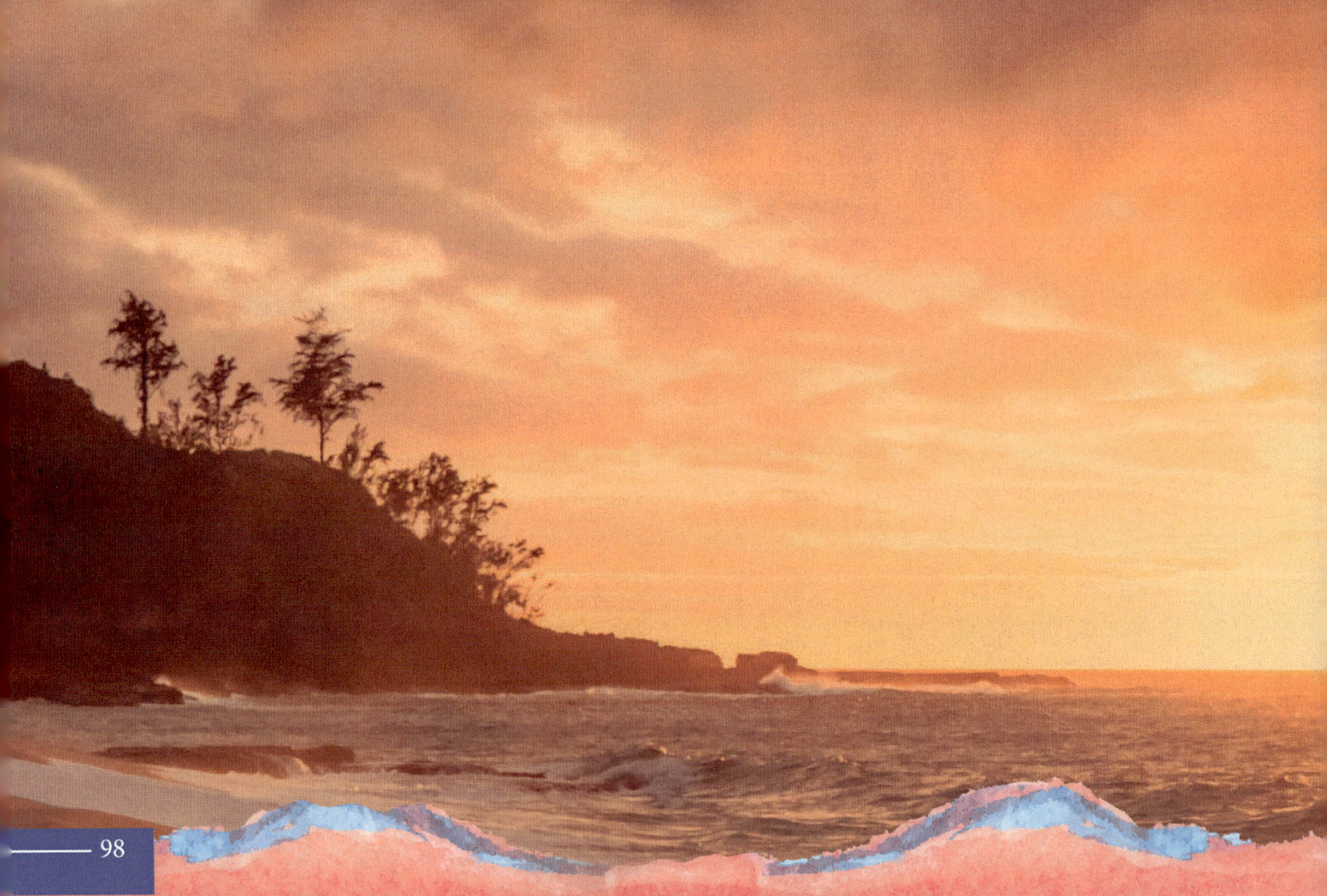

Concluding Thoughts

Let us conclude with this statement from the Book of First Thessalonians, chapter 23, verse 23 :

'May you be sanctified through and through, thoroughly. May your whole spirit, soul, and body be presented blameless at the coming of the Lord. And the One who calls you is faithful, and He will do it.'

Our hope is that this unveiling of the Word, will help you understand how you ought to participate in that which God intends to do in your life.

May grace and peace be your portion.
Amen.

Additional Resources

1. Website for Dr. Rani Samuel: **www.ranisamuel.co.za**
2. App for Dr. Sam Soleyn:
https://apps.apple.com/za/app/sam-soleyn-ministries/id1579794342

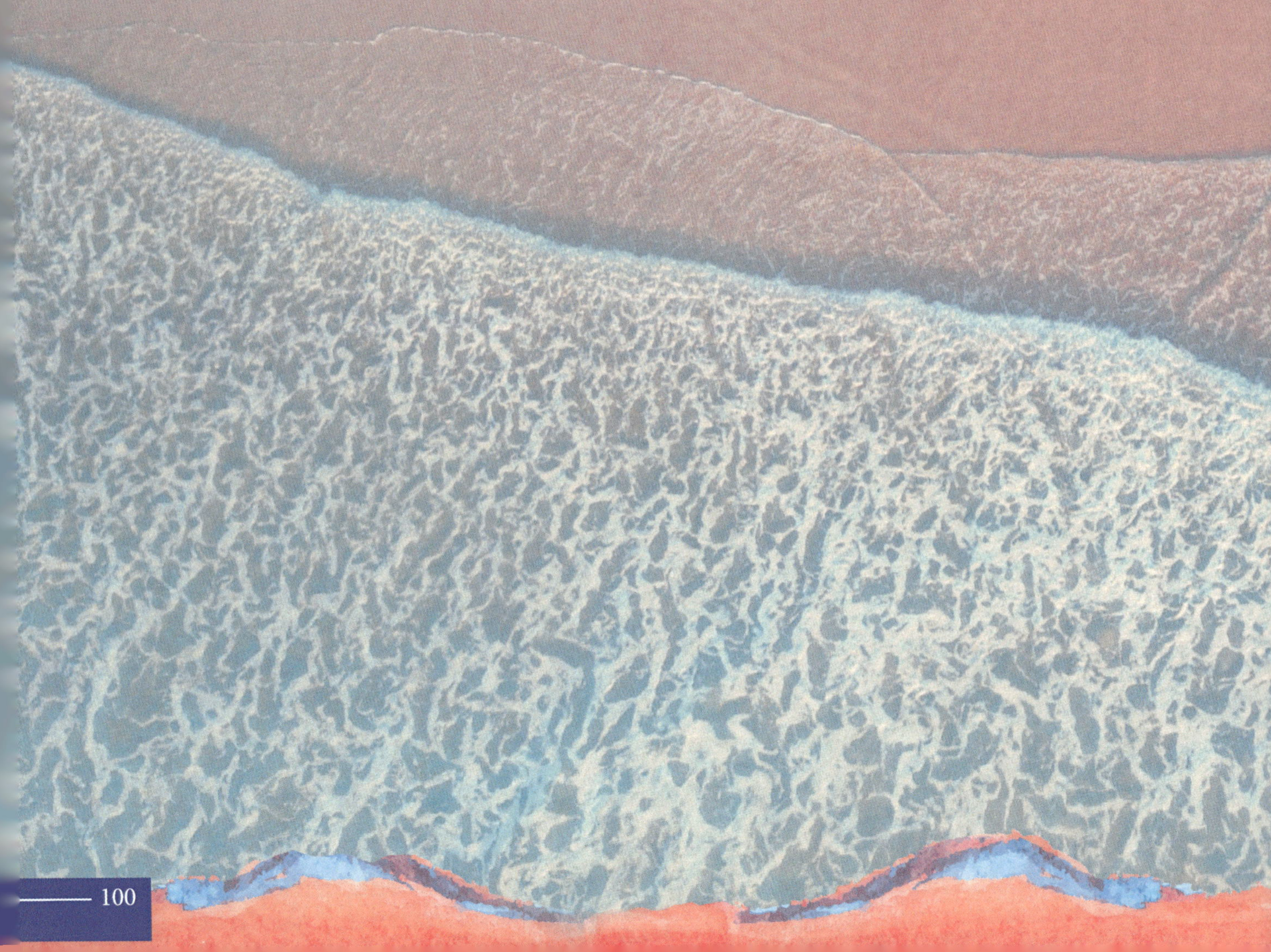

My Personal Journal

My Personal Journal

My Personal Journal

My Personal Journal

My Personal Journal

My Personal Journal

My Personal Journal

My Personal Journal

My Personal Journal

My Personal Journal

My Personal Journal